ORAL SEX FOR EVERY BODY

GIVING AND RECEIVING FOR MEN AND WOMEN

TINA ROBBINS

TRANSLATED BY TIM BARALIS

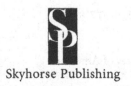

Skyhorse Publishing

Skyhorse Publishing books may be purchased in bulk at special discounts for sales promotion, corporate gifts, fund-raising, or educational purposes. Special editions can also be created to specifications. For details, contact the Special Sales Department, Skyhorse Publishing, 307 West 36th Street, 11th Floor, New York, NY 10018 or info@skyhorsepublishing.com.

Skyhorse® and Skyhorse Publishing® are registered trademarks of Skyhorse Publishing, Inc.®, a Delaware corporation.

Visit our website at www.skyhorsepublishing.com.

10 9 8 7 6 5 4 3

Library of Congress Cataloging-in-Publication Data is available on file.

Cover design by Rain Saukas

Cover photo credit Thinkstock

ISBN: 978-1-62914-476-4

E-book ISBN: 978-1-63220-077-8

Printed in the United States of America

Contents

INTRODUCTION   **7**

FOREPLAY   **9**
GOOD COMMUNICATIONS   9
PROCEED WITH CALM   10
USING ALL FIVE SENSES   11
THE ART OF CARESSING   13
TANTRIC MASSAGE FOR COUPLES   15
TURNING UP THE HEAT   16
TANTRIC CARESSES   17
AN ADDED PLEASURE   18
SAFE ORAL SEX   22

KISS ME AGAIN AND AGAIN!   **25**
SOUL KISSING   28
DEVOUR HIM/HER WITH DIFFERENT KINDS OF KISSES   29
DO YOU KNOW THE THREE P'S + C?   34
SKIN DEEP   34
YOU'VE GOT TEETH, USE THEM!   36
AN EXPLOSIVE PROCESS   37

SETTING THE STAGE   **39**
LOOK AT YOURSELF, LOOK AT YOUR PARTNER   39
THE POWER OF DÉCOR   40
SEXY UNDERTHINGS   41

Lingerie for All Tastes   42
Your "Down There" Look   42
The Scent of Sex   44
Tantric Aromas   45
The Feng Shui of Sex   46
Positioning the Bed   48
Breaking the Routine   50
Old Friends   51

Erogenous Territory   **55**
Skin   57
Hair   58
Eyes and Face   58
Lips   58
Neck, Nape, and Shoulders   59
Ears   59
Back   60
Rump   60
Arms   61
Wrists   61
Hands   61
Breasts   62
Abdomen   63
Navel   63
Crotch   64
Thighs   64
Ankles   64
Feet   64
Keep Touching Me!   65

Orgasm: An Explosion of Pleasure   **69**
The "G" Spot   70
Meeting Up in Phase Four   75

THE PUBOCOCCYGEUS MUSCLE:
  MORE INTENSE ORGASMS ... 80
"ORAL" ORGASMS ... 82
THE BENEFITS OF ORGASM ... 82

JUST ABOUT HER ... **87**
THE FEMALE BODY REVEALED ... 88
THE ART OF KISSING ... 94
CUNNILINGUS: ONWARD TO THE GRAND TREASURE! ... 96
THE BEST TECHNIQUES ... 98
OTHER RESOURCES ... 100
MASSAGING THE "YONI" ... 101

JUST ABOUT HIM ... **105**
CENTER OF HIS UNIVERSE ... 107
MASSAGING THE "LINGAM" ... 110
FELLATIO: MAKE HIM MELT WITH PLEASURE! ... 110
DIFFERENT FELLATIO TECHNIQUES ... 112
HOW DOES SEMEN TASTE? ... 115
TASTES AND SMELLS ... 116
TRICKS OF THE TRADE ... 117
ERRORS TO AVOID ... 119
GET COMFORTABLE ... 120

ORAL KAMA SUTRA ... **123**
POSITIONS FOR CUNNILINGUS ... 125
ADVICE FOR GUYS ... 130
POSITIONS FOR FELLATIO ... 133

RED HOT! ... **141**
INDECENT PROPOSALS ... 142
BREAKFAST IN BED ... 142
THE "BLACK KISS" ... 143
CHANGE OF SCENERY ... 146

HOW TASTY! 146
DOUBLE YOUR PLEASURE 148
THE MOST SENSUAL PIERCING 149
HOW ABOUT A SHOWER? 151
NAUGHTY PHONE SEX 152
DEEP THROAT 153
TWO FOR THE PRICE OF ONE 155
ORAL TANTRA 155

Introduction

When we are eating something we enjoy we often say: "This melts in your mouth." We are satisfied and we "savor" the experience. Enjoyment, savor, mouth, and satisfaction; I cannot find better words to begin this hopefully provocative guide about one of the most pleasurable sexual practices there is: oral sex.

Leave all timidity behind and prepare to take advantage of the most thrilling techniques, the most voluptuous kissing and caressing, all designed to drive your lover absolutely wild. This is a complete guide to learning how to both give and take, the most important aspect of oral sex being to join with your partner in climactic union, and getting there by engaging the five senses in a total communion.

Often we find ourselves burdened with inhibitions, taboos, or bouts of shyness, all of which hinder our relationships. If this is the case with you, then you have found the perfect book. Keep reading, and you will learn to free your body to go beyond your mental limits and completely enjoy an exciting session of oral lovemaking. Passionate sexual play enables us to explore our partner's body and feelings. It is a time for letting the imagination fly and for abandoning oneself completely to caresses, kisses, whispers, nibbles, and massages, all of which are part of the thrilling art of oral sex.

I will explain it all, step by step, without any hurry. Haste, indeed, is the worst enemy of sex. We are going to relish every moment, every gesture, each caress, allowing ourselves to unlock the most carefully guarded secrets of our deepest desire. Chapter by chapter we will go forward, sorting out the preliminaries, the different techniques (whether for him or her), different positions, the erogenous zones so enthralling to your lover, and a long list of fantasies and role playing which will enable you to enjoy sex as never before.

All will be presented in a form that is both pleasant and fun, for this is exactly what we are talking about: having great fun, and freeing oneself from hang ups, allowing yourself to be carried away by the moment. Oral sex is the most intimate and sensual form of contact, more so even than intercourse itself. To be brought to orgasm or to bring someone else to orgasm requires certain skills. No one is born with these skills and too many times we feel inhibited in communicating to our lover what we like or what excites us and ignites our passion. This play of strokes, rubs, kisses, wandering hands, lips, and tongue over the most sensitive parts of your partner will make your relationship much more fulfilling.

I suggest that you and your lover read this book together. I offer it for couples who wish to bring more creativity into their relationships, for self-conscious lovers who have yet to allow themselves to fully let go, for singles who want to try new things, and, generally, for all those who love good sex, in all its splendor!

Foreplay

Many couples believe that foreplay, that magic opportunity for seduction when the five senses begin to awaken sexual desire, starts with direct stimulation of the genitals, or, worse still, oral sex itself.

Oral sex, as its name clearly indicates, *is* sex, and therefore doesn't count as foreplay. Sure, sometimes you crave a "quicky," and this certainly can result in a satisfying experience. But, in general, a sensual and slow dalliance helps open up our senses as well as better prepare us for orgasm.

We are talking here about caressing, kissing, murmurings, erotic massage, which, by themselves, can make for fulfilling sex without the need for penetration. Sex based on these "preliminaries," without intercourse itself, is known as "petting."

GOOD COMMUNICATIONS

For starters, good communication, using both verbal and visual cues, is essential—just as essential as stretching out comfortably in the bed, turning off the lights, and letting go of any worries before getting started. It is important that each partner appreciates and praises the appearance and desirability of the other. It is the time to leave behind all fears of looking foolish and to break through any barriers of false modesty. Leave behind all taboos and prejudices, tell him or her what you like, what you want him or her to do, how he or she can give you more pleasure. Do this with words, looks, and little signals to indicate your wants and needs.

In the case of oral sex, fears and embarrassments often come up, which are easily overcome if we learn to communicate more clearly with our partner. There are men who love to get fellatio, but do not like to give cunnilingus, as well as women who feel ashamed to ask for it when the opportunity presents itself. It also happens that there are men who dive right into "69" without clearing it first with their lover. All of this provokes uneasiness which could be easily avoided with a simple look, gesture, or word.

PROCEED WITH CALM

In general, a man requires between two and three minutes of direct genital stimulation to achieve climax. This is not the case with the ladies, who need twenty to thirty minutes of sexual sport to reach orgasm. In addition, women usually require an extra dose of foreplay: kisses, caresses, sweet nothings, and glances make for a more fulfilling and satisfying act. We can employ any of these at any time during intercourse. Experienced couples know how to dole out these delights; they know when to hold back, they know when to speed up; they give them out affectionately as required to the different parts of their lover's body. The key is to *listen*, to *sense* your partner's desires and totally satisfy his or her need.

Haste can be the worst enemy of sex. Take your time. Savor the moment and relax. Anticipation is erotic and one of the most exciting factors in a relationship. Above all, avoid routines. There is nothing less exciting than a couple caught in predictability. Surprise your lover with new moves and different positions. Don't tip off your moves beforehand! Present your lover with new experiences. This is the best-kept secret to being a good lover.

USING ALL FIVE SENSES

Using our senses is the best aphrodisiac, as long as you don't squander the multiple possibilities they offer and discover the secrets of how to make the most of them.

Smell. This sense plays a most important role in sex, above all when it comes to oral sex. The human brain detects aromas, smells, and essences, which either increase or diminish the attraction between two people. The olfactory sense is powerful and very sensitive. It is the only sense that directly accesses the cerebral cortex; therefore, it is the quickest of the senses and determines, based on odor, whether we find another person attractive or not.

Smell operates differently in every person. What can excite one person can make another cringe. As in so many other things, everyone has their own preferences regarding smells.

But there is one thing on which all sexologists agree, and that is the important role pheromones play in sexual attraction. Every human body gives off odors. Some of them are perceived readily, such as the odor of sweat or the genitals. But there are others which elude the threshold of consciousness. Pheromones are part of this class of imperceptible odors. They are emitted by glands which are found in the armpits and around the sexual organs. Passing across the vomeronasal organ, which is located in the posterior part of the nose, pheromones trigger signals which go directly to the brain, where sexual excitement and attraction are produced.

- **Enticing aromas.** These are, par excellence, part of the erotic arsenal used in the sensual arts. You can choose among floral fragrances such as citrus blossom, bergamot, jasmine; fruit essences such as tangerine or lemon; exotic spices; sea scents made from fresh herbs; or musk perfume for men. Choose the one you like most, but remember, the natural scent of your body can also be very arousing, so don't overdo the use of perfumes.

If you prefer, you can also scent the room. For example, scented candles of ylang-ylang essence, sandalwood, and cinnamon produce bewitching effects on the sexual appetite. Try, also, different types of incense or simply put out a bouquet of fresh flowers. Use your imagination; sprinkle petals on the bed sheets and in the bath water.

Hearing. The sounds of pleasure. Learn to heed your partner's desires. His or her moans, breathing, and sighs are the best stimulants and an infallible guide for knowing what turns him or her on. Silent sex is liable to be very boring. This is not the time to be uptight. Whisper sweet words in his or her ear, cry out in pleasure, boss them around, beg them tenderly. Words can be a source of extremely pleasant arousal for our senses.

Sight. Turn on the lights. Set shame aside and let your partner behold you in your nakedness. Sex in the dark can often be very provocative, but there is nothing more exciting than to be able to see and touch each and every curve, bend, and corner of your lover's body. Watch how your partner gets excited, how he or she moves, how your partner touches him- or herself. Tell your lover what parts of his or her body you like the most. The room will heat up—count on it. Pay attention to your intimate apparel. There's nothing more sensual than a sexy ensemble of good quality. Let your partner kiss, caress, and *contemplate* your body.

Touch. Please touch. Caress your lover with the tips of your fingers, with your feet, with your thighs, with the inner part of your arms, with your breasts, with your tongue. Later I will explain the technique of how to give a good sensual massage.

Choose to make the bed with sheets of satin or silk. These are special fabrics whose smooth texture provides an added glamour and irresistible degree of sensuousness.

Taste. The taste of pleasure. Suck, lick, run your tongue over every inch of your lover's body. How does you partner's body taste? What do his or her lips taste like? Would you be willing to play with edibles such as honey or chocolate?

Remember, too, that many foods have aphrodisiac qualities: tomatoes, celery, figs, cacao, plantains, ginseng, nutmeg, and shellfish, among others.

According to research conducted by the Spanish Association for Sexual Health, a romantic supper is the preferred prelude to lovemaking favored by Europeans, and more than half of them invite their partner to dine with this end in sight. As you probably already know, sharing an enticing dinner can be the start of a great session of foreplay with an opportunity to introduce aphrodisiac recipes. Being mindful of this, remember that excessive alcohol consumption does not mix well with lovemaking!

THE ART OF CARESSING

Erotic massage is one of the most exhilarating forms of foreplay. It relaxes the muscles, dissipates tensions, calms the mind, and prepares us to totally let go in a session of torrid sex. It is an opportunity to share tenderness, affection, and unhindered skin-to-skin contact. Caressing is the most important element of foreplay.

The technique of erotic massage requires good timing and a calm approach. The ideal situation involves a quiet period of time when you won't be disturbed. Turn off the cell phone, make sure the thermostat is set to a comfortable temperature, around 75° Fahrenheit (25°C), and include, if it suits your fancy, some soothingly appropriate music, red roses, incense....

Aromatic oils and massage lotions will be your best friends. There is a huge range of choices available in the marketplace; just make sure that whatever you buy is quickly absorbable. Remember that creams take longer to be absorbed and can leave a disagreeable taste if, once the massage is underway, you wish to switch to using lips or tongue to stimulate your partner's body. So try pure oils such as olive oil, almond oil, and sunflower oil, all of which you can apply directly to the skin or mix with essential oils of sandalwood, ylang-ylang, patchouli, etc. If you want to make your own massage oil, it will suffice to add a couple of drops of essential oil to two tablespoons (30 ml) of any oil you use for a base. For mixing, it is better to choose an oil base that is odorless. Don't use virgin olive oil for mixing, since its odor is too strong and it doesn't mix well with the various essential oils. Besides, it will outlast any other aroma you happen to use.

Begin to undress your partner or have him or her do it themselves. The ideal position for them is face down with the head tilted to the side and arms half-bent at the same level as the head. It's important that your partner feel comfortable throughout the whole process. Cover the buttocks with a soft towel if he or she feels a little chilly at the start (the idea, however, is to get them warmed up in a hurry).

Since it is bound to be quite cold, warm a bit of aromatic oil in your hands before letting it contact your partner's skin.

Slide your oil-soaked fingertips over the skin of your partner's back and try out the following motions:

Circular. With the palms of your hands, employ different pressures on the back, making circles using a clockwise motion.

Sliding. Place your hands at the base of your partner's spine, with the fingers pointing upwards towards the head. Using your body weight, slide both hands along the length of the spinal column.

In our sexual massage, we can begin by caressing and gently rubbing the extremities, the hands, the feet, and the face. Later on, try out a gentle head massage. Pay careful attention to the back of the head, since it is extremely sensitive, and this way you will cause your lover to melt in ecstasy. Pay attention, as well, to the temples and crown of the head. Little by little we get into massaging the back, the neck, the shoulders, the legs. With the next pass we work the thighs, then inside the thighs, and then the breasts. And finally, the genitals.

Remember that you are not confined to using just your hands, but can also use such objects as feathers, a fringe, a silk handkerchief, etc. There are, besides, specific areas very sensitive to gentle rubbing, such as the earlobes, the cheeks, the neck and its nape, the inner part of the arms, the navel, the calves, and between the fingers and toes of the hands and feet.

You can also use your saliva and light blowing to cause differences in temperature on different areas of the skin such as the back or nape of the neck.

It's important that during erotic massage we avail ourselves of the sensations that are offered through the touching of our partner's body, exploring its curves, how it tenses here and there, its shapes, experiencing contact with the naked skin, taking note of the slightest details, while expressing complete gentleness and passion.

TANTRIC MASSAGE FOR COUPLES

If you wish to bring an exotic touch to your massage session as a couple, try out this pleasant ancient technique. Inspired by Hindu philosophy, it is a ritual of stroking the erogenous zones so as to achieve equanimity of spirit, as well as an orgasm which involves all the senses. For the one who practices Tantra, physical and sensory pleasures are the key to spiritual development; you can't have one without the other.

We can begin the session either standing or sitting face to face, totally nude. Here, also, it is important to have available a tranquil environment with soothing music and lit incense. We breathe slowly, giving full attention to our surroundings and all of our sensory impressions.

Touching the Roots. Anoint the feet of your partner with aromatic oil and massage them, pressing into and rubbing the muscles of the entire foot. Switch feet every two or three minutes.

Journey to the Privates. Using both hands, squeeze the thigh and continue upwards, very slowly, as far as the crotch.

Let It Happen. One of you relaxes an arm totally while the other massages it. Repeat with the other arm, then switch roles.

Spreading the Wings. The couple embraces and, each using both hands, kneads the upper region of the other's back from the shoulder blades to the neck.

Wave of Pleasure. Place both hands beneath the navel and slide them all over the solar plexus up to the shoulders. Then slide the hands all over the upper arm down to the hands.

Kissing the Chakras. Seated with backs pressed one against the other, each rocks the body gently, thereby experiencing the stimulating warmth of the spinal column. You will be surprised how exciting this exercise can be!

Final Relaxation. At the end of the session, both partners stretch out on the ground, facing each other with legs apart. She then places her legs over his legs. Next they grasp hands and allow the energy to flow between them. Breathing slowly, they reflect on all the pleasure they have just shared.

TURNING UP THE HEAT

A good massage, to be truly erotic and sensuous, cannot neglect the most sensitive and arousing zones of the body. Just remember that at this point in the process, we are not going for orgasm. If you see your partner is starting to get too excited, hold off from caressing them until they cool off a bit.

Pleasuring Him. With your partner completely undressed and lying on his back, kneel between his open legs. Rub a small amount of aromatic oil on your hands. Take his testicles in one hand and gently fondle them. With the other hand (well lubricated), stroke the shaft of his penis, starting at the root and going back and forth. Use the gentlest of pressures so as to induce greater excitation. With this massage, pleasure him with the aim of simply arousing him and not causing him to ejaculate.

Pleasuring Her. Ask your partner to lie on her back. Kneel between her open legs and place a small cushion beneath her knees so that she is comfortable. Do not apply any oil to her vulva. Instead, use a liquid sexual lubricant, which has been warmed by rubbing it in your hands before you start. Begin by gently caressing your partner's thighs, paying special attention to the inner parts of them. Continue, caressing her pubic hair and vulva with a gentle motion. Use your fingertips to lightly palpate the *labia majora* (big lips) of her vulva, maintaining a regular rhythm. With your other hand you can massage her breasts.

TANTRIC CARESSES

Tantric caresses are the best example of how one should start a sexual encounter. There are five phases of tantric caressing which, all together, should take at least an hour and a half to perform:

1. **Gentle Strokes.** Begin by caressing each other with gentle motions, starting with circles and then up-and-down patterns, for fifteen minutes. This is about slowly exploring the nooks and crannies of our partner's body, leaving the breasts and genitals for later.

2. **Silently Together.** Make him lie behind you, so as to enjoy the closeness of your bodies, but without getting too worked up. If the temptation is too great, then position yourselves face to face. Dedicate the next fifteen minutes to gazing in-

tensely into your partner's eyes and gently kissing their body. Maintain skin-to-skin contact. This is an opportunity to realize that an intimate relationship precludes inhibitions, blockages, fears, or shame.

3. Breasts and Genitals. Breathe gently, slowly, and deeply. The time has come to caress your partner's breasts and genitals with gentle circular movements, first with the hands close together and then moving them farther apart. Don't suppress any of your vocalizations; they too are an energy conduit and also a source of positive vibrations. Allow this phase to last for up to another half an hour.

Total Energy. Each partner now moves their hands up and down the genitals of the other. Rub along the entire length of his penis and make sure he touches your vulva with sensitivity, sweetly. Remain calm and patient; experience the totality of sensations as if time has stopped. Feel the sexual energy pervading your whole body, not just the genital area. To further this, it is good to run your hands all over your partner's back and spine, distributing that energy all around.

An Added Pleasure

Shared masturbation is one of the most thrilling and pleasurable forms of foreplay. In addition, combined with a hearty bout of oral sex, one can attain a very intense orgasm without the need for penetration.

The perfect antecedent to oral sex is masturbation. Gentle rubbing, the heavy breathing which comes close but doesn't touch, the first kisses, the tongue toying with our sex; these are most exciting preliminaries.

Remember that you should pace your seduction. Part of the success of your session relies on delayed gratification. If you notice yourself about to place your mouth on your partner's sexual part, stop, change your tack, and direct your attention to other erogenous areas on their body. Kiss the interior part of the thigh, caress their buttocks, have your tongue fondle the cup of their navel. Use your hands to rub between their gluteals, approaching the anus without touching it.

Pleasuring Him. In general, women prefer foreplay more than men. Men usually go straight for the "gusto." This happens mostly due to lack of knowledge or familiarity, but the truth is that once men discover what it's all about, they enjoy it just as much or even more than the ladies! The combination of amorous advances, rubbing, and caresses prior to engaging in fellatio can result in something very exciting that enhances the sexual encounter.

To reiterate: delayed gratification brings success. She can begin by kneeling at her lover's feet and rubbing her cheek against the bulging "parcel" in his pants, maintaining constant eye contact with him. Surely, he might want to go on the offensive, but this is precisely the moment she must take charge and decide the course of events. Massage his butt, his thighs, and the "bulge" waiting to be loosened from his pants. Carefully unbutton his trousers, lower his fly (you can even do this with your teeth), and let him keep his underpants on. Rub your hands over his briefs, massage his butt cheeks, nibble his thighs, play with his navel, but at no time make the slightest contact with his impatient "tool." Selfishly direct your attention to his legs, his inner thighs, the back of his knees, as well as his buns and navel.

Now fondle his balls and lift out his penis and stroke it with the ends of your fingers. Keep your mouth close to the glans (head of the penis), but don't touch it as yet. Men have a spot which is especially sensitive and can be stimulated to increase their excitement before oral sex. We're talking about the perineum, the area between the anus and sexual part (scrotum in men). You can stimulate it with two fingers, using alternating degrees of pressure over the zone.

Pleasuring Her. Start with a combination of kisses, humming, and fondles to clear the way for rubbing the pubis. With great delicacy, use your fingertips to press between the lips of the vulva. It is important to keep up a constant and gentle rhythm. While the hands and fingers are working on her below, run your tongue over her nipples, making circles around the areolas of both breasts on your way down to her belly button. Keep rubbing her carefully, until your tongue joins up with the fingers already there. Watch out for her clit! There are men who attack this most sensitive female organ in a rough and impatient manner. In general, women prefer that stimulation begin with the "hood" that protects the clitoris, going around it on the sides or underneath. While one hand is occupied with the clitoris, the other is free to stimulate her perineum (caressing, massaging, and pressing gently) and anus. Above all, it is important to maintain constant rhythmic contact so as to avoid putting the kibosh on her climax.

PROHIBITED ORAL SEX

Recently, the government of Singapore altered its penal code to allow the practice of anal and oral sex in this Asian country, though certain restrictions still apply. Both practices were legalized for consenting heterosexual adults in private. Certain associations favoring the rights of homosexuals vigorously protested, yet the law as written considers sexual relations between men to be a "transgression against the public morality."

Many women enjoy being masturbated during oral sex. Others even prefer to do it themselves, nudging their clitoris while their partner licks their vulva. Others ask their lover to put one or two fingers into their vagina during cunnilingus when they feel they are at the point of coming. And there are those who prefer to arrive at climax through intervention of the tongue alone.

A BIT OF HISTORY

In ancient Rome, to perform cunnilingus or fellatio was frowned upon. To receive either, however, was not an object of any reproach. One of the worst insults of that epoch was to accuse a man of giving fellatio to another man. Art has left us with examples of "prohibited" sexual acts eschewed by the Romans. One of the most extraordinary collections of pictures ever discovered is that of eight erotic vignettes located at a spa in the suburbs of Pompeii (Italy). In them one can behold all and each of the sexual taboos of the time: fellatio, group sex, cunnilingus, male and female homosexuality, etc. There is one image, however, which stands out as most scandalous. It depicts a woman performing cunnilingus on another woman who, at the same time, is performing fellatio on a man!

SOMEONE WRITES...

I've been with my present partner for twelve years now and our sexual relations are beginning to get somewhat "boring." Typically, when Saturday night rolls around, we jump into bed and almost by rote repeat the same positions, the same kisses, and the same words.

This went on until, one day, I made a decision and suggested something new to him. Both my guy and I love oral sex. So we started to do it in public places. The first time we did it in a subway car, early in the a.m., taking advantage of the fact that the car was empty. The next time was in a public park in plain daylight, we even did it in my office at work at closing time... Our favorite spot now is fitting rooms in the big department stores. It is so exciting that nowadays we hardly ever do it in bed. Really, our sex life has improved, big time!

Elisa, 34 years old

Safe Oral Sex

In the event you have oral sex with a stranger, or you aren't 100 percent sure about your lover's previous partners, it is recommended that you take preventative measures. A condom is the best way to avoid possible STDs (sexually transmitted diseases), and they come in a variety of flavors to boot. You can also use them to prevent the exchange of bodily fluids (one way is to cut the condom in half and place it over the vagina). You can buy female condoms, which prevent direct contact of the mouth with the vagina or anus. It is also recommended that if you are going to give fellatio to a stranger that you don't swallow his semen, and make sure that neither his pre-ejaculatory fluid nor semen enters your mouth, since this is considered a high-risk practice regarding the transmission of STDs.

An exciting way to practice oral sex is to put a condom on your lover using your mouth. Be careful using your teeth since these could damage the condom's material. This technique is ideal for the many men who lose their erection whenever they put on a condom. Oral stimulation will help prevent this undesirable letdown. To do this, put the condom in your mouth with the tip facing in the direction of your tongue. Then slowly, little by little, put it over his penis with your mouth, as if you were giving him a blow job, and push it down with your lips set against the rigid ring at the condom's opening. Throw away any condom you have used to practice fellatio; don't use it for intercourse since it is liable to have a nick or tear caused by your teeth.

During oral sex, not only is there contact with another's semen or vaginal fluids, but there is also the possibility of contracting a primary infection from blood. There might be a wound or open sore in the person's mouth which, if it starts to bleed, creates a risk of infection. Hepatitis B and AIDS can be transmitted this way, as well as through direct contact with someone's blood, and so it is not recommended that you have oral sex with anyone who has these diseases.

In general, almost all of the STDs, from genital herpes to gonorrhea, are capable of being transmitted by the mouth, and so it is best to avoid oral sex with someone if you suspect there is the possibility of contagion.

Kiss Me Again and Again!

In a book dedicated to oral sex you must have a chapter on the art of kissing. Giving and getting kisses anywhere on the body make up a great part of the erotic charge of the sexual act. A kiss is not just a means for getting sex; it is much more than that. A kiss is an erotic end in itself which can be just as exciting as intercourse. Kissing involves the senses of taste, touch, and smell—a combination of experiences which can turn kissing into an act of consummate provocation. Kisses can range from a fleeting, almost accidental brushing to those which signify a total physical merging via the lips. Between these two extremes lie numerous variations of kissing, though many people neglect this skill which, like any other skill, requires persistence, creativity, and patience to learn.

Surely you have, at one time or another, come across a lover who didn't know how to kiss. It seems to be a simple thing, but know-how is required to make it something pleasurable. A bad kiss can turn us right off; a good one can really set us ablaze. Here are some sure tips on how to make your partner explode every time you kiss him or her.

- **Good Taste, Good Smell.** Kissing is a very intimate act. Keeping this in mind, pay special attention to your oral hygiene so as to prevent bad breath. Keep some chewing gum or candy mints on hand to refresh your mouth in case you have just smoked or eaten something spicy. Make sure you wear good perfume or cologne, not just to avoid unpleasant body odor, but also to make the moment more inviting.

• **No Hurry.** Relax, breathe deeply, and enjoy the moment to the maximum. A kiss is an intimate and delicate act, so don't just push up against the lips of the other person in a rushed, abrupt way. Approach them tenderly, use sensuality to tempt them, and include love sounds which tell your companion just how much you are enjoying them. Remember that there is nothing more impersonal and cold than a kiss given with closed lips or open eyes!

• **Use Rhythm.** Kissing is a very intimate contact with your lover that should always be done with delicacy and softness. It is important to maintain this contact the whole time. You can start with a few slow kisses, gently, without much ardor. Then, no matter how much you turn up the heat, the total effect will be much more enticing if you maintain a sense of delicacy.

• **Don't Be a Bore.** Don't kiss the same way every time. Surprise your partner by being sensual and sexy simultaneously. You might start with long, slow kisses, with and without tongue. Toy with your lover's lips, suck them, kiss the corners of his or her mouth and caress them with the tip of your tongue without entering the mouth itself. Above all, give 100 percent. To kiss is one of the most intimate things there is. If you're not really into it, your lover will notice right away, and there is no bigger turnoff than that. You can't put too much emphasis on kissing. Caresses and sexual positions are important, but kissing is the foundation.

- **Four Kisses in One.** First just put your closed lips on those of your lover till he or she starts to shake, enraptured. Then swap saliva, using a nonchalant kiss which you then turn into something much deeper. Then put your tongue in your lover's mouth, and go for the most intense and penetrating contact possible. Finally, intertwine your tongues as deeply as you can.

- **Make Them Yours.** Use your hands to tenderly caress your lover as you kiss him or her, or just hold your partner tight. Use whatever look, murmur, or caress is at your disposal to intensify the moment.

- **The Open-Mouthed Kiss.** If you do this with moist lips, you will arouse thrillingly pleasant sensations in your partner as you proceed to caress the interior of his or her mouth.

- **What, Me Ashamed?** Kissing is a very sensual act, as well as something that frees you from bashfulness. Accompany your kisses with little whisperings, little touches, little grunts of pleasure. Your lips should be moist and open. In this way you will give him or her very exciting sensations as you continue to stimulate the inside of his or her mouth.

- **A Sensuous Vampire.** Gently and sensitively nibble your lover's lips. Then make them better with the moistened tip of your tongue. Your partner will burst with pleasure.

- **Your Seductive Tongue.** Both the tongue and lips are loaded with pleasure-sensing nerve endings, which can bring you all the way to orgasm. Take advantage of this by putting a hard tongue in your partner's mouth and moving it to and fro with a rhythmic, rubbing motion.

- **Play, Explore!** Run your tongue along the inside of your partner's mouth, introducing it between their lip and gums and massaging it. This will cause a thrilling tingle. You can also probe the bottom side of their tongue; nibble it, suck on it.

- **Working Together.** When one of you takes the initiative, the other should play along so as to increase the enjoyment. Block the movements of your partner's tongue, and then let it in willingly. Suck on it with light suction; this will turn your partner on and they will show you how much they like what you are doing.

SOUL KISSING

The tongue is chock-full of sensitive nerve endings. That's why soul kissing fires us up and is the best introduction to the sexual act. Below, I illustrate some techniques to enjoy this most pleasant and provocative kind of kiss.

Put your tongue in your partner's mouth and then nibble their lips, which are so close to yours. Put a bit more pressure on the lips so that the kiss turns into a light love bite.

Explore the interior of your lover's mouth with your tongue. Put it in the fold where the upper lip joins the gum and caress tenderly. Some people consider the tingling sensations this causes to be extremely exciting.

Explore the fold where the lower lip joins the gum. Then stroke underneath your partner's tongue as far back as the frenulum (tongue web). Savor it.

Form your tongue into a funnel; put it in your partner's mouth and move it in and out rhythmically. The friction of tongue and lips sometimes can have the same effect as the penis moving back and forth in the vagina; the difference being the lips and tongue are crammed with pleasure-stimulating nerve endings.

If you want to take this kind of tongue caress all the way, suck your partner's tongue until you sense his or her body getting totally into the action.

DEVOUR HIM/HER WITH DIFFERENT KINDS OF KISSES

Kissing is an erotic, sensual activity. As such, you must bring a dose of the pleasantly unexpected into the process that makes your lover melt in delight. If you want to mix up your kisses, here are some suggestions:

- **Exotic Kisses.** I'm sure you know about the Kama Sutra, but have you heard of the *Ananga Ranga*? Both contain similar ideas, though they were written centuries apart. Whereas the Kama Sutra was written for all types of lovers (married or not), the objective of the *Ananga Ranga* was to help spouses guard against boredom and tedium in marriage. Its pages are loaded with a refined eroticism, and it also pays special attention to women (something rare in that day).

An example from the *Ananga Ranga* is a kiss that shares its name and that consists of gently covering the eyes of your lover with your hand and placing your tongue between his or her lips. Then you run your tongue in and out of their mouth while they keep their eyes shut. Their temporary "blindness" will enhance experiencing the warmth of your breath and sweetness of your tongue.

On the other hand, the following types of kisses appear in the Kama Sutra:

- **The Bent Kiss.** This happens when the heads of the two lovers are tilted in opposite directions. It is one of the most common varieties of kissing and is the preferred type in the movies. Tilting the heads allows better contact of the partners' lips and profound penetration of their tongues. It is an excellent way to start a passionate love session and arouse your partner.
- **The Nominal Kiss.** When the lovers' lips just brush against each other.
- **The Throbbing Kiss.** When, with lips touching, the lovers move their lower lips only.

- **Touching Kiss.** This occurs when the girl brushes her lover's lips with her tongue, closes her eyes, and places her hands between his.
- **The Direct Kiss.** The lovers place their lips in direct contact and both move in a simultaneous rubbing. The important thing here is that they suck and nibble each other's lips, also caressing with the tongue. This is a long and relaxed kiss which can express strong passion, and one which excites a lot of people even more when the tongue is not used.
- **Gyrating Kiss.** This one involves the lover taking his or her partner and turning their face in order to kiss them on the mouth, while gently moving their own head from side to side.
- **Pressed Kiss.** The lovers kiss and strongly press their lower lips together. This kiss is used to either start or stop the loveplay; it's not convenient to hold it for a long time.
- **Kiss of the Upper Lip.** This happens when one of the lovers takes the upper lip of the partner with their teeth, and then the other lover reciprocates in turn, taking the lower lip of the first partner. In the Kama Sutra this is presented as if one of the lovers takes the initiative while the other passively responds. Perhaps this is due to the fact that the text was addressed to men as being active and women being passive. With couples of today, however, each one should be as creative as possible and give free reign to their imagination.
- **The Clasping Kiss.** Here, one of the lovers uses their lips to seize those of the other. When the one doing the kissing touches their tongue against the teeth, gums, tongue, or palate of the other, the kiss is called "the fighting of the tongue."
- **Kiss That Kindles the Flame.** This kiss is given on the corners of the lover's mouth in the middle of the night so as to awaken their affection.
- **Eyelash Kiss.** This is when you kiss your partner all over their face and then kiss their eyelashes.

- **Kissing with the Fingers.** Here the lover moistens the fingers of their hand, fingers kept close together, and then presses the hand on the mouth of their partner.
- **Traveling Kiss.** This is any kiss which your lover "blows" to you from a distance.
- **Nipple Kiss.** The kisses which work best on the nipples are those which are given gently, using a bit of saliva. Next, pressure is increased and, if the partner likes and wants it, one takes the nipple in their teeth and presses slightly. Some like to experience a twinge of pain there as they are about to orgasm.
- **The Timeless Kiss.** This involves total focus on the partner's body. The more you maintain control and the more you keep centered on caressing every part of the partner's body, the greater the intensity of the pleasure both will share.

KISSING IS HEALTHY

It has been shown that the act of kissing has a long list of benefits:
- It reduces both stress and accumulated negative energy. Kissing stimulates regions of the brain that release substances which give rise to the feelings of wellbeing. It is, in fact, an excellent anti-depressive.
- It stimulates the body's immune system. Kissing helps to fight illness.
- When we kiss, saliva production increases and this helps not only to eliminate bacteria in the mouth, but also to reduce the risk of cavities, gum disease, and bad breath.
- Kissing profoundly improves the muscle tone of the tongue and face and makes your skin appear much healthier and happier.
- A kiss releases adrenaline into the bloodstream, which improves the cardiac rhythm.

More Kisses. In his book *The Art of Kissing,* author William Cane describes different modalities of kissing. Here I show you some of his examples so that you can practice them with your lover:

- **The Tongue Kiss (or French Kiss).** This is about exploring the mouth cavity of the other person, but delicately.
- **The Clinging Kiss.** Here, one takes the partner's lips with his or her own.
- **The Opposite Directions Kiss.** Both lovers tilt their heads in opposite directions when they kiss.
- **The Vacuum Kiss.** Take one of your partner's lips (either the top or bottom) and suck on it.
- **The Tempting Kiss.** Kiss your partner without stopping until he or she can no longer resist.
- **Contact Kiss.** Brush your partner's lips with your tongue in the most cursory and light manner.
- **The Biting Kiss.** This one is about biting your lover's lips, but in a way that is both passionate and sensual at the same time, thus heating things up in the moment.
- **The Passionate Kiss.** In this type of kiss the excitement keeps mounting; both partners kiss each other, mixing tenderness with ardor, strongly pressing their lips together. Their hands also join in, each rubbing all over the other's body as they maintain the kiss.
- **Eskimo Kiss.** Gently touch the tip of your partner's nose with your own nose-tip. Then caress your partner's face with your nose-tip. This represents tenderness.
- **Pecking Kiss.** Kiss quickly, only with the lips and without using the tongue.
- **Sour Kiss.** Put a little lemon juice on your lips and kiss your lover passionately.

DID YOU KNOW....?

- We use more than thirty facial muscles when we kiss.
- According to a study published by Princeton University in 1997, the human brain is equipped with neurons which help one to find the lips of their partner with eyes closed or in dark places.
- The Bible is the first book to mention kissing, with forty references in the Old Testament alone.
- The most kisses given in a motion picture were delivered by John Barrymore in *Don Juan*—a total of 191 smooches.
- The longest movie kiss lasted three minutes and five seconds, shared by Jane Wyman and Regis Toomey in *You're in the Army Now*. And speaking of long kisses, the record is held by Dror Orpaz and Carmit Tsubara of Tel Aviv. In 1999 they lasted thirty hours and forty minutes with their mouths stuck together, after which they were taken to the hospital with serious facial pains.

THE TEN COMMANDMENTS OF KISSING

1. Don't think about anything except kissing when you're doing it. Better yet, don't think at all.
2. Relax your lips, but not to the point of drooping.
3. Kiss as if you had all the time in the world.
4. Use your hands. Increase pressure gradually and make sure to rub gently.
5. Don't turn every kiss into a sex act.
6. Always kiss your lover as if it were the first time.
7. Keep your eyes closed.
8. Two or more little pecks are a nice way to set up a big, hot smacker.
9. Enjoy a variety of short and long kisses before going on to little bites, little licks....
10. Make sure to end on a good note. An easy, sweet ending is much nicer than a curt, clangorous goodbye!

DO YOU KNOW THE THREE P'S + C?

To become a complete master of kissing, always keep the three P's + C formula in mind. We are referring to Patience, Passion, Pressure, and Calm. Kissing should always be a gentle, delicate, and unhurried act. Many men often abuse the French kiss by starting off way too forcefully, by jettisoning those little gestures and touches which lend so much pleasure to it. The French kiss isn't a battle of tongues, nor is it a way to choke your lover.

SKIN DEEP

Besides being your largest erogenous zone, the skin is also the body's biggest organ. For the average male its area is 20.5 square feet (1.9 square meters); for the average woman, 17.2 square feet (1.6 square meters). You can give a good kiss on the mouth or any other part of the body. The mouth is hot, moist, smooth, and sensitive, all of which turn it into a dynamite tool for pleasure. On the other hand, the tongue, together with the fingers is the most sensitive and deft part of the body. For this reason it excels when used to caress or massage. It is also central to the sense of taste and allows one, by probing the partner's body, to both give and receive pleasure.

Kissing, sucking, nibbling, and licking are all charged with passion and sensuality. They are all an art we need to learn if we want to drive our lover crazy with pleasure. A strong, passionate kiss can generate a multitude of sensations in both us and our partner.

After a kiss, the human body goes through physical changes such as shivers, heat, tension, and above all, sexual arousal. In women, a kiss, by itself, can even cause orgasm. Kisses are an open door to pleasure and enjoyment. A kiss gets the juices of sex and passion flowing. For this reason, whatever the form of sexual contact, whatever the erotic practice, kisses are essential.

One of the most exciting kinds of erotic kissing involves kissing the neck. It is important to give attention to this most erogenous of zones, particularly the back of the neck. Bite your partner's neck with passion and sensuality; run your tongue over it from top to bottom. Your lover will go nuts after a good session of neck kissing.

Another erogenous zone that is very susceptible to kissing is the ears, particularly the earlobes. You can practice nibbling and sucking the earlobes gently as you blow on them while you whisper dirty nothings in your partner's ear.

While you are kissing your lover's body, it is important that your hands never stop caressing its other points. The effect of both kissing and touching will ignite your partner's delight in the blink of an eye. And speaking of eyes, I'm sure you already know they are the "portals to the soul" and gateway to your feelings. Always maintain constant eye contact with your lover; this is the way to establish a more profound "chemistry" with him or her.

The breast is another extremely erogenous zone. With a woman, don't go straight for her nipples. It is better to approach them sliding your tongue down from her mouth by way of her neck while you grasp her waist with both hands. Then run your mouth over the curves of her breasts and kiss them, moving bit-by-bit closer to the nipple. Kiss the nipple gently, passing your moist tongue over its puckered surface while continuing to caress the rest of her body.

A man's nipples are just as sensitive as a woman's. The difference is that men are slower to respond to stimulation on them. To stimulate your guy's nipples, caress, suck, and lick them, just the same way you would want him to stimulate yours. Stretch them carefully with your lips, teeth, or fingers, and then release them. Go over them with a circular motion using the tip of your tongue and blow on them. Press down on them with your fingers, with your own nipples, or with your tongue. You can use other parts of your body to massage them and drive him mad with pleasure.

It's been proven that men like to kiss and caress this area much more than women like to receive such attention. This is because the area around the nipple (areola) releases a pheromone which increases the male's excitement. The funny thing is that men's nipples do the same thing, but, for some reason, few men consider this to be very exciting.

After stimulating your lover's nipples, you can gently move down towards his or her belly. Alternate your kisses with gentle strokes. As you kiss your partner, keep using your hands to massage his or her breasts or buttocks; just don't touch their private parts yet. If your partner is on their back, use a caress or gesture to have them roll over onto their stomach. Massage the spheres of their rump, starting out gently, and then finally ending in a crescendo of strong squeezes.

Are you aware that the nerve endings which lie on both halves of the back are extremely sensitive? Run your tongue over this area while you gently rub it.

Just like the hands, feet also are incredibly sensitive. So don't forget to kiss them and run your tongue all over them. As you do this, make sure not to cause any unpleasant tickling with your caresses.

Lick, kiss, nibble, and suck all those toes, from first to last. And don't forget the soles of your partner's feet; they are very excitable and a powerful erogenous zone.

YOU'VE GOT TEETH, USE THEM!

Biting is a very important part of the erotic tradition of India. The *Kama Sutra* offers us a fine list of love bites with a wealth of details:

- **Bite of the Boar.** This type of biting consists of making several rows of bold marks in rows very close together, with red intervals (like the footprints boars leave in the mud) between them. These bites are usually made on the shoulder.

- **The Broken Cloud.** This is carried out by making unequal ridges of skin in a circle, produced by biting with space between the teeth. The *Kama Sutra* specifies that this type of bite should be made on the breasts.

- **The Hidden Bite.** This bite is applied to the lower lip, leaving an intense, red mark.

- **The Swollen Bite.** This is produced when a large amount of skin is taken between the teeth prior to biting.

- **The Point.** In this instance, a small quantity of skin is grabbed by the teeth, leaving a mark that resembles a small red point.

- **The Line of Points.** A small portion of skin is bitten with all the teeth, leaving a line of their imprints.

- **The Coral and the Jewel.** This bite results from bringing the teeth and the lips together. The lips are the coral and the teeth are the jewel.

AN EXPLOSIVE PROCESS

During a high-intensity kiss, our organism goes through a chain reaction, beginning with an increase in the levels of dopamine (the substance associated with a sense of well-being) and testosterone (the hormone associated with sexual desire). Next, a series of glands secretes adrenaline and noradrenaline, which raise the blood pressure and heart rate. At the same time, the pituitary gland (situated in the base of the brain) releases oxytocin, also known as the "pleasure hormone."

According to the Kinsey Institute for Research in Sex, five of the twelve cranial nerves which determine cerebral function are involved in an erotic kiss, and due to the neural connections of lips, tongue, and cheek with the brain, a kiss allows someone to collect a lot of data about the other person, including their temperature, smell, and odor.

Setting the Stage

Spontaneous sex in unexpected places can be exhilarating and delightful. But with a little imagination, you can arrange an in-home setting for equally erotic, sensual encounters, without taking a step outside. Consider how environment with all its details is just as important to your lovemaking as the passion and creativity you put into every caress and movement.

LOOK AT YOURSELF, LOOK AT YOUR PARTNER

A good thing to do when setting the scene of your little love nest is to place one or more mirrors in strategic locations. Leave shame behind and enjoy watching your nude bodies as you engage in sex. Truly, there are few things more exciting than to watch the looks and reactions of your lover in plain view. You need only use your imagination. For example, you can pretend you are in public, or that the image in the mirror is a stranger watching you. If making love in front of a mirror bothers you, you can put on a mask, allowing yourself an anonymity which will let you reach new heights of uninhibited eroticism. This is also ideal for engaging in "solo sex." Masturbation can be very stimulating when you see the image in the mirror as *someone else* touching and pleasuring you.

The Power of Décor

Your surroundings play an important part in foreplay. Your favorite nick-nacks, gorgeous fabrics, and exotic colors will become the best aphrodisiac for your love-making. The idea is to come up with those appointments which encircle you in sensual and inspiring warmth. Consider, for example, how a minimalist or neutral décor can turn you off and chill your desire. The easiest thing to do to keep things on a high note is to experiment with the color of the walls. It's important to choose colors which agree with your personality. The secret is to cover one wall with the color you've picked and paint the rest of the walls with lighter tones of the same. Dark chocolate, cherry, or brownish-grey tones, for example, go with everything and are ideal for matching with items of bold, brilliant colors (fuchsia, red, turquoise blue, etc.), such as pillows, covers, candles, and carpets.

Another option would be to use wallpaper of a natural, pop, or classical, etc., motif.

There are many ways you can use interior design to achieve a more erotic ambience. I recommend that you create veils; experiment with the diaphanous properties of various materials so that you create an intimate, enticing space using lace curtains, Japanese screens, and exotic, semi-transparent curtains. The bedroom set, for example, hung with some gauze curtains (like you would hang mosquito netting or a canopy), will create a sensual, smashing effect.

Furniture also plays a part in creating an alluring environment in the home. Don't be afraid to try different things, to shake things up with different styles or formats. There is nothing more boring than a livingroom or bedroom where everything looks the same.

Comfort plays an important part in foreplay. Don't skimp when it comes time to decorating the house with warm carpets, fluffy cushions, velvet-covered furniture, crepe, big pillows...

Here are some other items which will provide an irresistibly aphrodisiac touch for your home:

Different-shaped mirrors. In the livingroom as well as bedroom, choose mirrors which are over-the-top, baroque, and glamorous. Ideally, you should place a large dressing mirror next to the bed so you can watch while you're making love.

Pictures and photos with erotic scenes and subjects. These will always be a suggestive accompaniment to your sexual play.

Crystal lamps are much sexier than the florescent type. Play with indirect lighting, dimmers, and all sorts of lamps of more personal designs.

If you have a terrace, paint it in brilliant colors. Fill it with plants and create a "chill-out" zone; include a hammock!

Experiment with candles and candelabra spread throughout the house. You can put little piles of petals around them, providing a wonderfully evocative touch.

For those marathon sex sessions, have at hand a tray of dried fruits, *baklava*, dates, *halwa,* and artisan teas.

SEXY UNDERTHINGS

It was Homer, in one of his tales, who told how Aphrodite leant her magic girdle to Hera, Zeus's wife, so that Hera could regain her husband's affection. It's possible that this is the first reference to the use of undergarments, which the Greeks and Egyptians considered an attribute of advanced civilization.

The role of lingerie is twofold. Firstly, it should make you feel like you're the sexiest and most irresistible woman on the planet, and secondly, it should wake up your lover's desire. Forget about having a perfect body. Your attitude, demeanor, and self-esteem are what make you sexy.

Take the initiative to wear more daring garments. This little "extra" will increase your partner's desire a thousand-fold, and why not choose the lingerie together? Let him give vent to his most hidden desires which haunt his heart.

Besides, the special fabrics used to make lingerie are quite capable of giving you any number of erotic thrills throughout the day, whetting your appetite for what is to come at night!

LINGERIE FOR ALL TASTES

Every woman has her own distinct and personal style, inside and out. The objective is to get whatever makes you feel like the most irresistible woman in the world, always true to your own self.

- **Romantic.** Wear bikinis and *tangas* with gaudy flowers, lace, embroidery, delicate fabrics, and pastel colors.
- **Elegant.** You can find lingerie of high couture and exquisite design, made of fabric bordered with silk that fits you like a second skin.
- **Sport-Chic.** Cotton is the perfect textile. Choose fun patterns with numbers, letters, lines, tropical flowers, or suggestive messages.
- **Innovator.** Dare to try out camouflage patterns, menswear, and outfits with military insignia.

YOUR "DOWN THERE" LOOK

In a book on oral sex, genitals are an important aspect. It's a sure thing you don't hesitate to depilate your bikini line when summertime arrives. Why stop there? How about showing your companion a new "shaved" look and cause him to blow his gourd? Most men find a woman's pubic area very attractive. The classic image is that of a triangle or simple vertical strip. Try something more daring, even edgy: totally shaved! This choice makes oral sex very enjoyable for both lovers when it's that "time to dive."

It used to be unthinkable that a man would shave his body hair, but every day we see more cases of depilated guys and we're not in the least surprised by it. Movies have had their influence on this "fashion" *(Basic Instinct)* and even some television shows *(Sex in the City)*. The absence of down (on both pubis and penis) allows for unique and much more intense sensations. That being said, the main requirement for this new style is for him to shave very closely. You should be aware, however, that when shaved, this area will be more exposed to the downside of over-zealous rubbing and, for women especially, beard stubble can cause nasty, stinging, beard burns.

If you're going to go for a shaved bush, keep the following in mind:

- **Shaving the pubis and/or genitals** requires hygienic conditions so that harmful bacteria don't penetrate the skin.
- **Use properly sterilized tweezers and scissors** before you begin any depilation. If you're going to cut your pubes flush, avoid razor contact with the skin. If you cut yourself, use a disinfectant immediately.
- **Don't use the same razor** for different sessions or different areas of the body. Shaving with a used blade can cause infection; besides, it's liable to be rusty.
- **The pubic area is very sensitive.** Be careful using waxes, creams, or gels, which can cause harm to the skin. Test the product before you use it.
- **Soak your pubes under the shower** with warm water before removing them.
- **If you experience irritation,** stop and wait until it dies down. Take time for your skin to adjust to the shaving process.
- **After you're done,** moisturize the area with a good moisturizing cream.
- **There are beauty parlors** that specialize in this type of hair removal.

If you would like to share the shaving ritual with your lover, you can turn it into something playful and sexy. Have your partner gently apply moisturizing cream on your body with gentle strokes. Next, use a soft brush to apply shaving cream to the area to be shaved (up, down, and on the sides), slowly and carefully. Shave. The hairs will "bite" a bit as they are removed; this is why you should use moisturizing cream. If you intend to keep the area shaved, re-shave every two days so that the hairs don't get too long and you avoid the sting of shaving them. Use a gentle touch. If you feel daring, you can depilate your entire body!

THE SCENT OF SEX

Pheromones are those odorless chemical substances capable of waking the sexual impulse in both humans and animals.

The word itself is derived from Greek: "pherein" means to carry, and "horme" means an impulse, i.e., something which excites.

Pheromones normally accumulate in the skin and are released into the air. Minute amounts of pheromone, when inhaled, produce potent substances which provoke very intense reactions.

Pheromones are released by glands found in the armpits and around the sexual organs. Passing over the vomeronasal organ (VNO), located in the nose, pheromones cause signals which are routed to the brain, and it is there that our human experiences and reactions are formed. There are two human sex pheromones: those secreted by males (androstenone) and those secreted by females (copulin).

Today you can buy products that contain synthetic pheromones with the aim of making us more attractive and alluring. There are perfumes, shampoos, shaving creams, condoms, body lotions, seasonings (for food), and even men's handkerchiefs impregnated with this sexually stimulating substance.

It is also possible to increase the supply of one's pheromones using completely natural means. Here are a few suggestions:

- **Maintain regular sexual relations.** Having sex at least once a week will cause an increase in pheromone production.
- **Practice oral sex.**
- **Exercising** helps stimulate the apocrine (sweat) glands which are producers of pheromones. Sports activities produce profuse sweating, which boosts production of these beloved chemicals.
- **Avoid using deodorants** with strong perfume, since these neutralize the effectiveness of your own natural fragrance. It is advisable to use deodorants, which block perspiration but don't eliminate your own sexual scent.
- **Don't be too quick to remove** fresh sweat from your body, unless there's too much of it or the odor is disagreeable.

TANTRIC AROMAS

The Tantric path of the East recognizes the power that human pheromones have regarding seduction, whether giving or receiving it. Sex is viewed as a path to enlightenment, and all aspects of Tantric ritual are regarded as fundamentally important. Beyond the sexual act itself, Tantra deals with the increase of desire and passion. For this reason, we are urged not to suppress our body odors excessively with colognes and perfumes, since this is liable to thwart desire. The aromas of sweat and the secretions of the sexual organs are alleged to be potent aphrodisiacs.

With regard to aphrodisiacs, different authors who specialize in Tantric sex invite us to use any number of natural aromas to strongly excite the passion of lovers. They recommend using incense and essential oil heaters to perfume the room where you are going to make love.

These perfumes include:

- **Basil.** Basil's powers are well-known in many Eastern cultures. Place a small plant of it in your room or heat some drops of its essential oil.
- **Sage.** Known since ancient times, it is recommended to burn some dry leaves of sage to affect an immediate aphrodisiac response.
- **Cilantro.** Grind some seeds into a powder and mix with musk and saffron to obtain a wonderful incense.
- **Jasmine.** This is a much-used ingredient in essential oils for massage. In the East, where its characteristics are well-know, it is often used to scent the bed of newlyweds.
- **Lily.** To obtain its stimulating qualities burn some dried flower in the room. This will guarantee a high degree of sensual pleasure.
- **Vanilla.** For the Pre-Colombian Indians, vanilla was an aphrodisiac considered worthy of the gods. It has a sweet, subtle, but penetrating odor.
- **Ylang-ylang.** This is an exotic Eastern oil that is sweet and penetrating.

THE FENG SHUI OF SEX

This ancient art, based on how energy flows in the interior of a house, can also help in sexual matters. The idea behind it is to create harmonious surroundings where attraction, eroticism, tenderness, and sentiments contribute to the fulfillment of the relationship.

Feng Shui bases its efficacy on working with the presence of the Five Elements of Nature (Earth, Water, Fire, Metal, and Wood) in the home.

EARTH

- **Is associated with** fertility, motherhood, and home atmosphere.
- **Attracts** stability and security in relationships.

- **Is reflected in** stable, tender relationships.
- **Is evoked with** yellow and brown walls and fabrics.

WATER

- **Is associated with** adventure, freedom, and deep thinking.
- **Attracts** excitement, independence, and communication.
- **Is reflected in** a deep sexual relationship, full of feelings, but little passion.
- **Is evoked with** fountains, aquariums, and mirrors.

FIRE

- **Is associated with** spontaneity, joy, and passion.
- **Attracts** bipolarity of feeling and sentiment.
- **Is reflected in** sexual unions full of ardor, though short-lived.
- **Is evoked with** candles, orange colors, brilliant reds, and yellows.

METAL

- **Is associated with** harmony, clarity, and romance.
- **Attracts** clear thoughts and feelings.
- **Is reflected in** a sincere sexual relationship that is open and direct.
- **Is evoked with** articles and sculptures of metal, circular forms, greens, and blues.

WOOD

- **Is associated with** candor, momentum, and creativity.
- **Attracts** direct, guileless communication.
- **Is reflected in** sexual affairs full of ups and downs and sudden turns.
- **Is evoked with** anything made of wood.

POSITIONING THE BED

With the aim of achieving surroundings charged with eroticism and sensuality, Feng Shui offers a few key points when it's time to choose a bed and how to position it in the lovers' room. Here they are:

- Avoid placing the foot of the bed at a door opening. This will tend to precipitate nasty, continual arguing.
- The distance between the bed and any window should be enough to preclude distraction, supporting a sense of spaciousness.
- It is important that the headboard be of solid wood and that it doesn't shift during lovemaking. This reinforces a feeling of mutual trust.
- The bed should be somewhat higher than normal, which will insure that the couple's sense of oneness is put on a firm footing with a strong emotional bond uniting them.

COLOR IS IMPORTANT

- **RED.** Energy, passion, love, and power. This color furthers excitement and fantasies in bed. That being said, lovers who love red are usually quite domineering and possessive.
- **ORANGE.** Joy, creativity, warmth, and cordiality. Along with red, orange is the color of sexual passion.
- **YELLOW.** Mental clarity, energy, and purity. This color suits calm lovers, those who are conventional in their sexual relationship.
- **GREEN.** Hope, health, fertility. Those who prefer this color are open and innocent in their approach to sex. In surroundings of this color, however, there can be a noticeable lack of passion.
- **BLUE.** Tranquility, honesty, and freedom. This color invites delicacy, affection, and tenderness. It is ideal for first dates.

- **WHITE.** The color of purification and spirituality, prohibited for devotees. This color is for insipid lovers, those who prefer to make love with the lights out, using the missionary position.
- **BROWN.** Intimacy, sensitivity. This color is ideal for leisurely, deep, and long sessions of lovemaking.

SOME CURIOUS FACTS

La Federación Española de Sociedades de Sexología (The Spanish Federation of Sexology Societies) has recently conducted an interesting study to find out about the attitudes and sexual practices of Spaniards. Here are some of the findings:

When it comes time to choose where to make love, Spaniards overwhelmingly (66%) admit to using the same spot they always use.

The place they prefer, by far (94%), is their own home. The bedroom is the favorite place (93%), followed by the den (24%), the bathroom (13%), and, curiously enough, the kitchen (9%).

Among those who prefer to conduct their amorous encounters outside the home, the car is the location chosen by the majority of those surveyed (11%), followed closely by hotels (10%), the beach or country (8%), and, finally, the house of a friend (4%).

Regarding the environment where the sexual encounter takes place, it is curious that although more than half of those surveyed (51%) consider surroundings to be very important and prefer them to be special, their actual conduct does not follow their stated preference. More than half of those surveyed in the sample (52%) said they pay no attention to their surroundings during sex!

In contrast to this, there are the 45% who actually take care to ensure an ambience that makes the evening something special. The elements most used for this are: background music (55%), candles (36%), drinks (19%), and special attire (19%). At the bottom of the list are erotic movies (6%) and cuddling (1%).

BREAKING THE ROUTINE

In this chapter, we have been dealing at length with the subject of the home setting. But what if you opt for a different location—somewhere more exciting?

Get a hotel room with your guy in the middle of the week. Keep it a secret; invite him for what appears to be a simple dinner date or drink in a hotel bar. When he arrives, take him directly to the suite. Pick a hotel with class, meet him wearing your sexiest outfit, and buy him a gift. If you want to make it more mysterious, send him a text message with only the address of the hotel and the room number. When he arrives at the scheduled time, greet him at the door with a glass of champagne in your hand, naked!

Another hot idea to change the setting is to take advantage of when your best friend is away on a trip and ask to borrow her apartment. Once you're sure the flat is totally at your disposal and you have the keys in hand, call your man and tell him you want to make crazy love with him. Tell him you have a place where you are going to keep him "captive" without interruption.

The idea of having sex on someone else's bed, sofa, or carpet will delight him. If you make the "show-no-mercy" tone of your invitation convincing enough, you will get his erotic juices flowing and he'll be ready to share a sensational sexual soiree with you, pronto.

To close the deal, you can also offer him a little weekend trip.

Sex outside the home is always a wonderful way to experience the thrill of something new and break up the routine. If it is not always convenient to find the time or pretext for such an adventure, make sure you keep this as your "plan A" for those emergencies when you need to jump-start your partner's sexual appetite and creativity.

Once the bags are packed and you are on your way, worries will dissipate with every passing mile.

To plan a spur-of-the-moment escape, you need only four things:

1. Rental or use of a cabin in the country. You don't need anything fancy, just a little bungalow out of the city.

2. A strong urge to get away and make passionate love.

3. A toothbrush and clean set of undies.

4. To convince your partner this weekend will be unlike anything else, that you don't want to spend it watching TV. Follow your impulse to escape the city noise, without an itinerary. This is usually the best way to go.

OLD FRIENDS

We've already talked about the importance of imagination in foreplay with your lover. And while we're on the subject of play: there's nothing better than a good collection of toys to play with. Sexual toys, that is....

Don't kid yourself that sex toys are a new idea. They've been around for over 2,500 years. The ancient Egyptians and Greeks were already using dildos, as well as the Romans. Ancient Chinese manuscripts explain how to tie a silk scarf at the base of the penis in order to maintain an erection (primitive version of today's cock rings).

Some of these aids were quite imaginative: the Chinese "porcupine" consisted of a circle of fine feathers attached to a silver ring, which was fitted over the penis.

We can engage in oral sex using some of these toys as pleasant accompaniments. For example, you can introduce a dildo into your partner's anus while you lick her clitoris. Or, you can put the dildo into her vagina while you give her the pleasure of a "black kiss," that is, lick her anus. The possibilities are endless.

You can even buy a chin-strap dildo as an aid to oral sex, using it to penetrate your lover while you perform cunnilingus on her.

Another popular sexual toy that is ideal for oral sex is "Chinese" or Ben Wa balls. These are also known as "Geisha" balls and they come in several varieties, for insertion in the vagina or anus, or "punishment balls" which are spiked (soft rubber) for added stimulation. They are also available with an internal vibrator. All are ideal for providing an extra treat for your lover during a session of oral sex.

The balls used for insertion and stimulation of the vagina are the "original" Ben Wa balls. They contain a smaller ball inside, which produces added excitation to the vagina when the balls are moved.

The balls used for anal stimulation are smaller than the ones used for the vagina and they have no smaller ball inside. They are placed in the anus one at a time, dilating and stimulating the anal opening. Later they are removed one by one, producing exquisite pleasure. There is a form of these comprised of balls on a string. They can be used to stimulate the anus of both men and women. Remember that any penetration of the anus must be undertaken gently, and if your partner is not used to this sort of thing, it is a good idea to use very small balls with a liquid lubricant especially formulated for anal use, so that the anal mucosa are not irritated.

The Ben Wa "punishment" balls have a surface full of protuberances, resembling small spines (non-injuring), which produce major stimulation and great increase of pleasure.

SOMEONE WRITES US...

I love the idea of being watched. One of my sexual fantasies was to do it with my boyfriend with someone else looking on. I didn't push this on him, but it so happened that one day, by coincidence, my hot fantasy was fulfilled. It happened when one of my friends was going on a trip to the United States and she asked me to take care of her plants while she was gone. The first few days I went to her apartment by myself and, while I was watering the plants on her terrace, I noticed a young man of about twenty-five on the other side of the building, paying close attention to my movements from behind a curtain.

His presence excited me and got my imagination going. At the end of the week I invited my partner over to my friend's place. It was summer. It was hot on the terrace and I suggested to my guy that we get naked to take in a little sun. Of course, I knew that young neighbor was watching us. Actually, he had been there every day watching me from behind his curtain.

I began to get really aroused and I pounced on my boyfriend. We did it a number of times without stifling any of our cries of passion. The neighbor couldn't believe what he was seeing and this turned me on even more. Before my girlfriend returned, I made sure we engaged in a couple of repeat performances. I will bet anything that neighbor will never forget me....

Joana, age 31

Erogenous Territory

So far, we've covered foreplay, caresses, sensual massage, all sorts of kisses, a setting loaded with pheromones, candles, and music, and then some. Now it's time to get down to the real deal and explore the pleasure regions which, when stimulated the right way, make every sexual encounter especially thrilling and memorable. Of course, we are talking about the erogenous zones, the best ticket to an intense, pleasurable climax.

Distributed over the entire body, the erogenous zones contain the greatest concentration of nerve endings. With sufficient stimulation, these nerve endings send a torrent of pleasure signals and sexual excitement directly to the brain. That doesn't mean, however, that this is an automatic process which works the same way in all individuals.

These "hot spots" are definitely affected by feelings and what goes on in the mind. That is to say, when your lover is in a state of high anticipation, any touch on his or her body is liable to cause a strong sexual response, since then all of their body is effectively one big erogenous zone and they are receiving contact from someone sexy to them. Everyone is different regarding their response to stimulation of the erogenous zones. For this reason, it is not a good idea to get hung up on what any sex manual says about how to excite your lover. The *entire* body, naturally, reacts in a positive way to sexual contact and stimulation.

In general, we are receptive to a great variety of stimuli: tactile, visual, verbal, etc. It's quite possible that what drives one person crazy with pleasure, say rubbing their neck or armpits, will turn someone else totally off. For this reason it is essential to have good communication with your partner. Not all of us are psychics. It works best if we "guide" our lover and show him or her what works with us, and what doesn't.

Most of us possess a long list of other places besides the genitals where we can experience erotic stimulation. There are many people, in fact, who have a special fixation on one of those other places. We find that if we concentrate solely on one of those areas, forgetting about the rest of the body, we can induce an effect equal or greater than direct stimulation of the genitals.

This is when we must engage our curiosity. Foreplay consists in exploring, trying different things, questioning, suggesting alternatives, etc. It means to go beyond any pre-established sexual conventions. Sometimes we get caught up in a tendency to be too restrained and unimaginative. That is the worst enemy of being a good lover. There is nothing less enticing than a predictable, monotonous, and boring sexual relationship. Sex is fun, passion, giving and taking pleasure, and should be without taboos, shame, or inhibitions. Many couples stick to making love with the genitals alone, taking the "fast track" to the one goal in mind: orgasm. It would be better if they learned to explore other possibilities that could give them even more pleasure.

In this regard, you should keep in mind that touch and sight are the principal senses. Looks, caresses, and rubbing—these are what create the conditions for thrilling sexual sport. Be naughty and start by leisurely taking off your partner's clothes. Remember that half-dressed is often more exciting than full nudity. Do a little striptease; wait until your lover is burning with desire, and then continue to enflame his or her desire until they can't see straight anymore!

Remember always, a good lover enjoys giving pleasure as much as receiving it. The more you enjoy delighting your lover, the better you will get at doing it and the more he or she will enjoy it. Do everything with enthusiasm, never mechanically or premeditated. Explore new territories and try new approaches; change intensities. This way you'll know what works and what doesn't. In every sexual relation, it is vital to be aware of what we are doing and what responses we elicit. It is a matter of watching for cues: listening to their grunts of pleasure, their cries, and observing their facial expressions and glances while you are covering their body with caresses, kisses, and hot licks.

Skin

With 2,700 square inches (18,000 cm^2) of skin and close to a million and a half sensitive nerve endings, the skin is the erogenous zone par excellence, and, beyond a doubt, the most extensive. We've already discussed the importance of touch in sexual relations. Desire and excitement arise due to sensory signals that arrive at the brain via the skin. Stroking, kissing, and massaging the skin are the best prelude to sex—a total gift to our senses.

The stimulation of this organ represents one of the principal driving forces of sexual activity. In addition, just looking at the bare skin of your lover or contact of naked skin between two lovers can ignite profound passion. Even so, sexual response to these stimuli (mostly visual) is more rapid in men than in women.

Hair

One of the first steps in sex is getting your partner to relax. Many times we jump into sex after a hard day at the office, still burdened with business concerns and stress. More than likely we find ourselves somewhat blocked, and we are not yet at that point of relaxation needed to enjoy a good love making session.

To start by rubbing and massaging your partner's scalp produces very pleasant relaxation and is the best way to both start and end our sex play. We can use our thumbs to give our partner a nice massage, making sure not to forget their temples and forehead.

In a moment of heightened excitement, we may even grab our partner's hair more aggressively, being careful, however, not to cause them any pain or injury.

Eyes and Face

Sight is one of the best aphrodisiacs there is. Visual contact reinforces the intimate connection of the moment. Forget about turning off the lights and doing it in the dark. Look straight at your partner; bring your lips close to him or her, and delicately kiss their half-closed eyelids. Continue by kissing their cheeks with delicate tenderness. Do this all over their face. Feel their body temperature rise. Rub the back of a hand or a finger over their face. Start with the chin, the cheeks, and later downwards to the neck. Do this sensitively, with feeling.

Lips

Obviously one of the most erogenous zones, the lips are perfect for giving and receiving sexual pleasure. We've already talked about the erotic power of kissing in previous chapters. Do not skimp when you kiss, and accompany your kisses with licks, nibbles, and sighs, which make your lover dissolve in ecstasy.

Try not to be so predictable. Surprise your partner with kisses on his or her body in places where he or she is unaccustomed to being kissed. Cover your lover with your lips, with your tongue, with your saliva, and with your breath. Don't forget to use your hands while you're kissing, gently stroking your partner's hair, face, back, etc.

The upper lip and the area between it and the nose are particularly susceptible to erotic stimulation. Approach them delicately and slowly. Take turns kissing first the upper lip and then the lower one. Use your tongue to moisten all around their lips. Another fun thing to do is to touch tongue tips with your partner.

Neck, Nape, and Shoulders

I'm sure you have shivered as your partner nibbled your neck and ran his or her warm breath over your skin. Psychologically, the one who allows their nape to be massaged is demonstrating trust in their partner, and the one who is doing the massage is showing their tenderness.

While you kiss your companion's neck, run your fingers through his or her hair, over their ears, and other parts of their neck. Make sure your lips are always a little bit wet; just don't slobber.

Ears

These are among the most sensitive parts of the body, and those who think otherwise usually have the most sensitive ears of all! For both sexes, the earlobes and back of the ear are particularly sensitive. To stimulate the ears, use your lips, tongue, and fingers.

You can try the following technique: put the tip of your tongue inside your partner's ear and make little circles. Then lick the earlobe and take it between your lips, grasping it gently. Repeat this over the other parts of their ear and alternate caressing with lips and tongue. You can blow on their ear from behind. If you add some sweet words and sighs to this, I guarantee you will cause him or her to melt. Remember that while your mouth has fun with your companion's ear, your fingers can join in, playing with the ear and hair as well.

BACK

Along the spinal column there is a string of very sensitive nerve endings. Using massage and stroking to stimulate them (always use up-and-down movement) will cause a hot sensation of pleasure to course through your partner's body. The flanks of the back respond, most of all, to delicate passings-over of the tongue and fingertips.

You can also run the tip of your tongue all over your partner's back, or do the same with little kisses, starting from the nape of the neck and proceeding down to the rump. Precisely there, right at the sacrum, is a very responsive area, just where the back connects with the gluteals.

Massages on this area are the most enjoyable and provocative aspect of foreplay. Try rubbing your body with oil and use your body to massage your partner all over his body. Run your slick breasts all over his back, his butt, and his abdomen. Move seductively and rub his genitals until he bursts.

RUMP

The rump is one of the most sensitive erogenous areas of a woman, especially when it is massaged using a lifting and separating movement. During oral sex, she will totally enjoy it when you massage her butt cheeks and scratch them lightly. The upper area of the butt, specifically the part which joins the back, is particularly sensitive, especially in women. Massage your partner there and watch as the tensions in the back dissipate, permitting increased blood flow to her sexual organs.

ARMS

The armpits, above all (be careful not to tickle them), and the interior surface of the upper arms are the most erotogenic points of the arms. When it comes time to stimulate these most sensitive areas, remember that it will excite your partner more to use strokes or kisses rather than pressure and massage.

Continuing downwards, we eventually come to the hands. These have more than forty thousand nerve endings which we are certainly not going to overlook!

Put your partner's hand on your mouth and run over it with the tip of your tongue. This provokes an unusual and exciting sensation. Equally exciting is another technique involving tracing little circles with your fingers, starting in the center of the palm, and spiraling outward. Go up and down them, making gentle strokes.

WRISTS

Though these are likely to escape the notice of lovers, they too have their place. To discover it, have your partner place his or her hands palms up and touch their wrists with your fingertips. After you stroke them a bit, use your lips, teeth, and tongue to lightly lick and nibble the center of one of them. You can kiss your partner's wrist with the palm of their hand on your face.

HANDS

Try stimulating the palms of your partner's hands using this seductive massage: have him or her face their palms up, and rub their wrists with your fingertips, along with their forearms, all the time whispering words of love to them. After a few minutes of this, use your lips, teeth, and tongue to lick and nibble the center area of their wrist. Hold your partner's hand, keeping it against your face.

BREASTS

Without a doubt, breasts are one of a woman's pleasure centers. Men, too, respond to stimulation of their breasts, though with less intensity than women. You can massage, stroke, kiss, or lick them; there are unlimited ways to pleasure your partner's breasts. You can also use *your* breasts to massage different parts of your lover's body. One exciting way is to take the man's penis and put it between both breasts, masturbating him by keeping constant pressure on his penis with vertical movements until he orgasms.

The nipples, as well, are extremely susceptible to stimulation, equally for men and women. You can blow them, suck them, pinch them gently, or squeeze them between your lips while you touch them lightly with your tongue. They are also a clear indicator of our level of excitement. When sexually excited, the nipples secrete oxytocin (the hormone of love) and become erect. Many people, especially women, can reach climax through stimulation of this area alone.

In general, men tend to treat this area a little brusquely, especially when they are nearing maximum excitement. The nipples are extremely delicate, and aggressive stimulation of them can cause discomfort, and even pain.

Here is a good way for a man to control over-enthusiastic sucking: place a grape between your teeth and move it with your tongue. When you can do this without breaking its skin, then you can say you have mastered the correct pressure you need to apply to nipples to pleasure them.

ABDOMEN

We have here another promising erogenous zone (especially for men), due to its proximity to the genitals. For men, the area between the navel and pubic bone is eminently susceptible to caressing and responds with intensity to all stimulations.

Draw a vertical line with your tongue, fingers, and lips, going from the navel to the pubis. Trace another line, this time horizontal, from one hip to the other and cover it with kisses, with the tip of your fingers or fingernails, subtly, without causing irritation to your partner. Accompany these with light sucking and nibbles.

Another suggested way to stimulate the abdomen is to put your hand about a half-inch (1 cm) above its surface, creating a pleasant experience of static electricity. Your partner will sense the warmth of your hand. When he least expects it, slide your fingers over his belly. When he closes his eyes, concentrate on the lower part of his belly and stroke it with a small brush, your makeup brush for example, and brush him in unexpected places. One of the easiest ways to get your partner going is to use ways of stroking and caressing that are well out of the ordinary routine. You can try using handkerchiefs of soft silk or feathers.

NAVEL

Due to its closeness to the genitals, this is one of the hottest areas of the human body. Stimulating it first provides the best beginning to oral sex. This might cause tickling, but applying strawberries, whipped cream, or an ice cube, for example, immediately transforms this contact into a "must" of our sexual repertoire!

CROTCH

Especially sensitive in men, use your fingers to gently massage from the hip to the inside of the thigh. If you combine this with oral pleasuring in the direction of the genitals, it will provide a greatly sensual start to oral sex.

THIGHS

The interior part of the thighs, where the skin is smoothest, is susceptible to being a great source of pleasure if it is properly stimulated with strokes, licks, or kisses. Try to rub it using a circular motion. Avoid nibbling this area, as it will leave noticeable marks. Keep away from the genitals. The more you apply oral pleasure here, the more it will excite your lover.

Another surprisingly sensitive part is the backside of the knees. When your partner is lying on their stomach, you can take advantage of this and use the tip of your tongue to go over them. Some advice: don't nibble or press your tongue with too much pressure. This area is much more responsive to gentle attention.

ANKLES

Place your lover's ankles on your thighs and rub them vigorously with your hands, working back towards the knee. Then kiss them on both sides. Make little circles on them with your fingers to add to the enjoyment.

FEET

Just like the hands, the feet contain great numbers of nerve endings; do not forget to include them in your sexual fun. Go all out with sensual sucking, licking, and little nibbles.

A good round of sex for both partners could include using feet to play with the other's genitals. If you do this, however, be careful. It is more difficult to control the movements of the feet than the hands.

KEEP TOUCHING ME!

We've already commented on how touch is a primary sense when it's time to give and take pleasure during foreplay.

Massage is a seductive way to kindle those erogenous zones.

Chinese Erotic Massage. Chinese erotic massage is based on the belief that the body's energy field is maintained by twelve "meridians," which channel the sexual energy and thereby increase well-being. To give a Taoist massage to your partner and introduce them to new sensations, have them stretch out, face up. Sit at the top of their head, either on your ankles or squatting.

Stretch your partner's skin from head to hips, taking it between your thumb and index finger and tugging it with gentle little pulls at every point.

Then, starting at the inside of the ankles, rub your fingers up your partner's leg slowly, from the calves to the thighs.

Place your hands together in the center of your lover's sternum and, very slowly, slide them down in the direction of the pubic bone. When you get to the hips, let your hands separate, rubbing over them; then return up by way of the sides to the armpits, then up over the chest and back to the sternum.

Keep repeating this movement, descending a bit more each time, until you are rubbing the genitals and getting close to the nipples on the return circuit. Trace a semi-circle on your part-ner's thigh, starting from the inside of the knee and going up and then down over the outside of it.

To end, use your thumbs to make little circles on the inside of his or her ears.

To become an expert in Chinese erotic massage, it is important to learn to manipulate your hands using a series of effective and pleasure-eliciting movements. The main ones are:

- **Drumming.** Close your fists and simply let them drop without using force. Increase the cadence more and more rapidly. Applying these vibrations will increase energy flow.

- **Hand Rubbing.** Fully extend your hand. Put it on the area you are going to treat, and press with the lower phalanges (small bones) of the hand. Don't lift your hand; it works best with gentle sliding.

- **Rubbing with Fingertips.** Extend the fingers of the hand. Place your fingertips on the desired area and slide them with sure firmness.

- **Finger Pressure.** Put your middle finger on the place to be treated. Put the index finger of the other hand on the middle finger. Slide the middle finger firmly and slowly.

- **The Pincer.** Make a pincer with the thumb and the other fingers of the hand. It's important to keep the other fingers together tightly. Gently grab the chosen area and stretch the skin outwards, again gently. Once you've stretched the skin, hold it for a count of twenty. Repeat this ten times for every place you massage.

- **Laying On of Hands.** Stretch out your hands and place them on the area to be treated.

- **Nail Massage.** Place the nails of your hand on the area you've chosen. The palm of your hand should be facing up. Slide the nails back and forth using a smooth motion.

- **Circular Massage.** Place the index and middle fingers close together on the area to be treated and rub lightly. Then, press more firmly.

TEST. WHAT DO YOU LIKE MOST?

To enjoy sex it is important to know your body well, what makes you feel sexy, and what parts, when stimulated, drive you wild.

Complete the following test and discover which of your erogenous zones are the hottest. We've left out the genitals which, obviously, are the primary pleasure areas and well-known as such.

If you have a companion, take the test with him or her and you will learn new things about them. If you do this, pay attention to the results and put what you learn into practice the next time you make love. (0=uncomfortable; 1=no sensation; 2=some pleasure; 3=a lot of pleasure; 4=orgasmic)

Lips	0	1	2	3	4
Face	0	1	2	3	4
Ears	0	1	2	3	4
Neck	0	1	2	3	4
Breasts	0	1	2	3	4
Nipples	0	1	2	3	4
Armpits	0	1	2	3	4
Arms	0	1	2	3	4
Hands	0	1	2	3	4
Thighs	0	1	2	3	4
Back	0	1	2	3	4
Rump	0	1	2	3	4
Feet	0	1	2	3	4
Fingers	0	1	2	3	4
Abdomen	0	1	2	3	4
Navel	0	1	2	3	4
Crotch	0	1	2	3	4
Nape	0	1	2	3	4
Shoulders	0	1	2	3	4
Hair	0	1	2	3	4
Skin	0	1	2	3	4

Once you know the most erotic zones of your body, you can begin to discover how you like to be stimulated on those areas. Remember, not everyone is a psychic, and to prioritize your zones will result in better communication with your partner. End of test.

WHAT DOES YOUR LIST LOOK LIKE?

In a recent Internet survey taken by women, the following results were obtained regarding their most erogenous zones. From least to most, these were their preferences:

10- Inner thighs	5- Feet
9- Back of the knee	4- Wrists
8- Butt	3- Breasts and nipples
7- Nape of Neck	2- Vagina and clitoris
6- Ears	1- Lips

Make your list and let your partner study it in detail. To discover and map your partner's erotic zones might take some time, but it will surely yield its rewards on the field of Eros. To be sure, this is a map which can never be totally finished. Depending on the situation or person involved, our bodies are capable of reacting in very different ways to sexual stimulation.

Orgasm: An Explosion of Pleasure

Good or bad, or simply different; quick (sometimes only seconds) or long-lasting; single or multiple. It's complicated to put all aspects of orgasm into words.

Orgasm is the cherry on top of the cake of a sexual encounter. It is sexual climax which can make us burst with pleasure. It is a physical chain reaction (mental, too) whose cause has not always been clear, especially when it comes to female orgasm.

The confusion started with the "Father of Psychoanalysis," Sigmund Freud, whose categorization of female orgasms provokes controversy to this very day. According to Freud, female orgasms are divided into two types: vaginal and clitoral. He considered clitoral orgasms to be a simple "intermediate" stage of pleasure, whereas vaginal orgasm represented a woman's reaching a "true" climax. One theory which Freud left in the background was the extremely important role the clitoris plays in a full sexual relationship.

This erroneous idea of two types of orgasm held sway until biologist Alfred Kinsey observed how important the clitoris was to female pleasure. After talking with thousands of women, Kinsey demonstrated that there was no reason to consider coitus as the easiest way to cause a female orgasm.

Later on, it was Masters and Johnson who emphasized the importance of the clitoris. After observing almost fifteen thousand instances of coitus and masturbation, the researchers came to the conclusion that there was just one type of orgasm, regardless of the means by which it was obtained.

These results were later supported by another prestigious investigator, Shere Hite. In her two reports on female sexuality (published in 1976 and 2000), it was stated that more than 70 percent of women surveyed stated that they did not arrive at orgasm by way of vaginal penetration without simultaneous stimulation of the clitoris.

THE "G" SPOT

It had been clear that the "star" of female orgasm was the clitoris. That was until 1950, when a German gynecologist named Ernst Gräfenberg discovered a small erogenous zone located in the vagina behind the pubic bone, near the urethra, about one-and-a-half to two inches (4 to 5 cm) back from the vaginal opening. He had discovered the now famous and controversial "G" spot. He did not delay in demonstrating that its direct stimulation provoked intense erotic excitation and pleasure in a majority of women.

It was sexologists John Perry and Beverly Whipple who, years later, actually named it the "G" spot, in honor of its discoverer. They concluded that in the vagina there was a place "extremely sensitive to firm pressure," which under adequate stimulation succeeded in triggering serial orgasms. In addition, Perry and Whipple brought to awareness the existence of female ejaculation and the relationship between the strength of a woman's pubococcygeus muscle (PC muscle) and her capacity for orgasm.

They quickly published a book that explained the results of their investigations and rapidly sold out in bookstores all over the world (it was translated into over twenty languages).

According to these investigators, there are three types of female orgasm:

- **Clitoral Orgasm.** Characterized by involuntary, rhythmic contractions of the pubococcygeus (PC) muscle. Penetration isn't required; only clitoral stimulation is necessary.
- **Uterine Orgasm.** This takes place as a result of deep penetration. This doesn't provoke multiple orgasms (as does clitoral orgasm), but the resulting single orgasm is very deep. This type of orgasm is not common.
- **"Mixed" Orgasm.** A combination of the two previous types. It is also know as vaginal orgasm or "G" spot orgasm. It is associated with contractions of the PC muscle characteristic of clitoral orgasm and the deep sensations of uterine orgasm.

In the case of men, two types of orgasm are described: one produced in the penis and the other in the prostate.

Since its discovery in the '50s, the "G" spot has been surrounded with controversy. Denied by some and defended by others, it has given rise to much contention among sexologists, doctors, and investigators throughout the whole world.

The latest revealing data about its existence came about thanks to research done at the University L'Aquila, in Italy.

In the study, there were nine women who claimed to have experienced vaginal orgasm or "G" spot orgasm, and eleven women who denied having them.

Body scanners attached to the participants showed that the tissue situated between the vagina and urethra (the place other studies designate as being the probable location of the "G" spot) was much more dense in the group experiencing the orgasms than the group that didn't. This would prove, according to the researchers, that the "G" spot is real.

Scientists of the Italian university concluded that a thicker vaginal wall close to the urethra can be linked with the presence of the contested "G" spot.

Locating the "G" Spot. It is not easy. The best way is to try to find it on your own, calmly exploring your own body, and once you find it to enjoy stimulating it. You can also use a vibrator (there are ones specifically designed for the "G" spot) to turn on this little treasure. Don't get bent out of shape if you don't find it the first time. This is totally normal, and the majority of women who never discover it at all find they don't need it to feel sexually fulfilled and complete.

Let's go through a series of steps to facilitate finding your "G" spot:

1. **Sit relaxed.** This is the ideal position, since if you are lying on your back it becomes harder to locate since gravity tends to pull your internal organs downwards (away from the vagina).

2. **Lubricate your fingers** with saliva or a bit of massage oil and gently stimulate your clitoris. It's important to keep the vagina excited and well lubricated in order to stimulate the "G" spot. Don't hurry; take as much time as you need.

3. **Introduce two fingers into the vagina** (ring and middle fingers). To help you know exactly where, first be aware that the Gräfenberg (or "G") spot is a small area located in the female genital area behind the pubic bone and near the urethra. So that there's no misunderstanding, let's imagine the face of a clock, centered at the vaginal opening. With the "12" pointing at the navel, the "G" spot would be located between twelve and one o'clock. Keep your fingers arched and make a tapping movement (not penetration). Do this rhythmically and continuously. When doing this, make sure your hands are completely clean and your nails are short; it would also be a good idea to use a little massage cream or oil to help the fingers fit inside.

4. Continue moving your fingers into the interior of your vagina. Imagine there is a kind of egg resting on the bottom of the vaginal wall. Use your fingers to go around this "egg." If you notice a swelling here, it means you have found your "G" spot.

5. Move one or two fingers over the area. Keep going over it; have fun with it. Now bend the finger(s) upwards and a bit to the left. The position of the fingers is very important when locating and stimulating the "G" spot. Notice how it swells up, how it throbs, and begins to feel good.

On the market there are vibrators designed specifically for stimulating the "G" spot (s-shaped dildos, also vibrators with a wide head). If you want, you can also have your partner search for your "little treasure." To do this, lay on your bed face down with your legs apart and your hips slightly elevated. Your partner should sit behind you and stimulate your clitoris using fingers, or, if you prefer, mouth or lips. This is a matter of starting slowly, bringing you to the point, bit by bit, where you are fully lubricated. When you are ready, ask your partner to put their fingers in your vagina, with the palm facing down. The idea is to explore the anterior wall of the vagina, maintaining firm pressure.

Meanwhile, move your pelvis so as to help your partner make contact with the "G" spot and describe what you are experiencing as it is stimulated.

It is possible to stimulate the "G" spot using fingers or tongue, combining the pressure of pushing down on the clitoris while simultaneously arching the tongue or finger upwards in a gentle, knocking movement. This should be done with the inserted finger from one to three inches (2.5 to 7.5 cm) inside the vagina to be effective.

Nevertheless, every woman probably needs a unique way of being stimulated. According to those who support the existence of the "G" spot, stimulating it will precipitate a vigorous, satisfying orgasm and will cause female ejaculation.

OTHER EROGENOUS SPOTS

The "G" spot has garnered all the fame, but there exist other highly erotogenic spots in a woman's genitals. If we learn how to stimulate them (orally or manually), we can experience intense and varied orgasms.

- **THE "A" SPOT.** This is located in the back of the vagina, about three-quarters of an inch to one and a quarter inches (2 to 3 cm) before the cervix and a bit behind the "G" spot. To stimulate it, slide your fingers half-way down the posterior wall of the vagina. There you will find an area that is bigger and slightly rougher than the rest of the vaginal wall. You are now at the "A" spot. It is stimulated virtually the same way as is the "G" spot. With this spot you can set off multiple orgasms (once you've reached maximal vaginal lubrication).

- **THE "K" SPOT.** It is located at the end of the vagina, just before the cervix. It is stimulated only by penetration; the penis must enter the vagina extremely deeply to reach it. The ideal position to do this is the man face-to-face with the woman. The woman lies on her back and puts her legs over the shoulders of the man.

- **THE "U" SPOT.** This spot is located near the urethra (through which urine is passed) beneath the clitoris. Oral stimulation is very pleasant here. To do it, put firm and constant pressure on the urethral area with the lower lip and teeth while touching with the tongue all over the area. One can also separate the *labia minora* (little lips) of the vulva to totally expose the urethra and caress it gently with the tongue.

They Have a "G" Spot Too!

It is none other than the prostate, one of the most inaccessible but, at the same time, most erogenous areas of a man's body.

The prostate is a small gland (resembling a nut) situated under the bladder and crossed over by the urethra.

To stimulate it, it is necessary to introduce a finger into the man's anus. It is here that we might meet with some resistance. Stimulating this area often causes men discomfort. It is best approached with great delicacy and, even better, when he is excited to the max. Lubricate your finger with some petroleum jelly or massage oil and slide it in gently. Pay attention to your guy's facial expressions and adapt your approach in accord with his reactions.

This works best with the man on his back and his legs drawn back as far as possible against his chest. This facilitates putting your finger in his anus (about two inches [5 cm]). You will find the prostate here by pressing in the direction of the penis. Gently massage the gland and the area around it. You can also pressure the prostate or lightly move your finger in and out to bring about orgasm.

Meeting Up in Phase Four

Sexologists agree in dividing the cycle of sexual response (for both men and women) into four phases: excitation, plateau, orgasm, and resolution.

Her Orgasm. The excitation phase of a woman, depending on several mental and physical factors, is usually accompanied by specific physical responses. The typical ones in this phase are:

- Start of vaginal lubrication.
- Expansion (by two-thirds) of the interior of the vagina.
- The *labia majora* (big lips) separate and the *labia minora* (little lips) increase in size (two or three times normal size).

- The clitoris grows in size and becomes erect. Just before climax the hood of the clitoris draws back.
- In this phase the clitoral glans is still not visible.
- The nipples may become erect as a result of muscular contractions. In addition, the breasts grow in size (approximately 25 percent larger).

During the plateau phase, a woman may experience the following:

- Increased vasocongestion of the vagina, which causes the outer third to swell. As a result, during this phase, the vaginal opening dilates.
- Vaginal lubrication diminishes, especially if this phase is drawn out.
- The *labia minora* (little lips) increase in size and their color changes considerably. They go from a pink shade to a more intense red.
- The clitoris becomes erect and the clitoral glans retracts towards the pubic bone and becomes more hidden behind its hood.
- The breasts increase in size, becoming 20 to 25 percent bigger than normal, and the area around the nipples (areola) also starts to swell.
- Many women experience sexual blushing in this phase as a result of increased blood flow in the skin's capillaries. The heart rate increases.
- A marked increase in muscular tension in the thighs and buttocks appears in this phase.

We now come to the orgasmic phase. In it, a woman may experience the following reactions:

- Rhythmic muscular contractions in the outer third of the vagina, womb, and anus. The first contractions are usually the most intense and occur every 0.8 seconds. As the orgasm continues, the contractions become less intense and more random. A moderate orgasm usually produces between three and five contractions, while a strong one can yield between ten and fifteen.

• The clitoris contracts considerably and the *labia minora* fold over and cover it.

• The blushing of the skin increases, covering most of the body.

• Muscular contractions are not limited to the pelvic region and may involve the whole body. Some women experience spasms in the back, hips, hands, or feet.

• During orgasm, some women emit a clear fluid from their urethra which is known as "female ejaculation" and is completely normal.

• In the final moments of orgasm, the entire body can become momentarily rigid.

During the final phase of female sexual response (resolution), a woman may experience:

• One or several more orgasms running through the body if stimulation continues.

• The vagina and its opening return to normal size.

• The nipples, lips, clitoris, and uterus return to their usual size, position, and color.

• Little by little the heart rate decreases and blood disperses from the genital area. This phase takes longer in women (it can take up to a half-hour for the clitoris to completely lose its erection).

• The sexual blush disappears from the skin.

• All of the musculature relaxes; the vaginal orifice and anus regain their normal tone.

In the event there is no orgasm, the woman experiences all the changes and reactions mentioned above, but at a much slower rhythm. As a consequence, blood engorging the pelvic organs may produce a sensation of heaviness and discomfort, due to its not having been released during the muscular contractions of orgasm itself.

His Orgasm. Now we will talk about masculine sexual response. It shares the same four phases, but with different physical reactions and its own rhythm.

During the excitation phase, a man experiences the following changes:

- Increase in blood flow causes the penis to become erect, and the skin reddens. This sexual reddening usually begins in the lower abdomen and spreads to the chest, neck, and face. It can also appear on the shoulders, forearms, and thighs. After orgasm, this blushing disappears more quickly in men than in women. It disappears first from the shoulders and extremities, then the chest, and finally the neck and face.

- A man's breasts also respond to sexual arousal. Frequently, a man's nipples will swell and become erect. This occurs without direct stimulation and can last up to an hour after ejaculation.

- Heart rate increases; the respiratory rate accelerates and blood pressure goes up.

- During the excitation phase, the man's scrotum becomes denser along with the testicles (up to 50 percent more). The testicles cling to the perineum, indicating imminent ejaculation.

Arriving at the plateau phase, the man experiences the following reactions:

- The penis attains its maximum erect size.
- The testicles rise considerably.
- Close to orgasm, the man is hit with the feeling that ejaculation is inevitable. From the first appearance of this sensation there is a brief interval of two to three seconds, during which he feels ejaculation is imminent and cannot be stopped, put off, or controlled in any way. This experience of inevitability of ejaculation takes place as the seminal fluid concentrates in the urethra of the prostate, just before it's actually emitted. Though the female orgasm can be interrupted by external stimuli, male orgasm, once started, cannot be stopped until ejaculation is complete.
- Before ejaculation, the glans may change color. Also, a drop of pre-ejaculate fluid may appear at the urethral opening of the penis.

The orgasm phase in the man is quite evident as it coincides with ejaculation, but there are other reactions as well:

- Along with emission of semen, four or five rhythmic spasms of the prostate, seminal vesicles, and urethra occur.
- During orgasm, the penis contracts in a way similar to the vagina's contraction during a woman's climax.
- Just as the female experiences, men have involuntary contractions of the inner and outer anal sphincters. These contractions occur every 0.8 seconds.
- Heart rate and blood pressure increase.
- This phase can last between three and thirty seconds, depending on intensity. The contractions start in very short intervals and, after three or four forceful expulsions, both frequency and capacity to expel quickly decrease.
- Light residual contractions may continue with minimal expulsion of seminal fluid of little or no force, lasting a few more seconds and occurring irregularly.

- In general, men find an abundant ejaculation more pleasurable than one of less volume. That's why pleasure may be greater with an ejaculation that occurs after a prolonged period of holding back rather than with repeated orgasms. Curiously, this is the opposite with women. The majority of women experience more pleasure with the second or third orgasm than with the first.

We finally arrive at the phase of resolution, which in men is characterized by the following physical reactions:

- After ejaculation, the penis becomes flaccid. There is then a recovery period, which lasts from a few minutes to several hours, in which the man cannot have another ejaculation. Women, on the other hand, do not experience this recovery period and are capable of successive and multiple orgasms.
- The sexual blushing disappears and a light sweat may appear on the skin.
- Once the penis has returned to its normal size, the man relaxes and often feels sleepy.
- The testicles and scrotum descend anywhere from five to thirty minutes after orgasm.

THE PUBOCOCCYGEUS MUSCLE: MORE INTENSE ORGASMS

The name is quite clinical, but this small muscle is capable of affording us greatly exciting and pleasant orgasms. But, where is it? Here, we're dealing with the principal muscle of the pelvic floor which extends from the pubic bone to the lower part of the back. There is an easy way to locate it. It is the muscle we contract when we try to either interrupt or hold back urinating.

This muscle is quite sensitive, being connected to the pelvic nerve, a branch of which connects the uterus with the bladder in a woman. For this reason, a simple contraction of the PC stimulates the pelvis, the vagina, and the uterus, making it a great ally for female sexual pleasure.

The pubococcygeus is a voluntary muscle, which means we can move it whenever we want. As such, we can train it using specific exercises to improve the quality of our orgasms.

Kegel exercises (named after Arnold Kegel, who developed them to control urinary incontinence) are very simple to do and involve tensing and relaxing the PC, in sets of repetitions, in order to increase its tone and strength. It is recommended to start out slowly with fifty reps a day and gradually increase the number up to two hundred per day. You contract and release the muscle, just as if you were holding back the urge to urinate. You can do this anywhere, anytime: watching TV, sitting in your office, on the train, etc.

On the other hand, the PC is an excellent ejaculation stopper. If you're in the middle of oral sex and you see your partner is ready to come and you want to keep stimulating him a while longer, you can do this using the pubococcygeus. All you have to do is stop stimulating him and press his PC for a few seconds.

The Kegel exercises also are ideal for improving a man's erection. While they tone the muscles of the vagina, Kegel exercises also facilitate an increase in blood flow to the penis, which improves erections and increases optimum control over ejaculation.

KEGEL EXERCISES...

...TO STRENGTHEN THE PENIS:
- Contract the PC muscle for three seconds, as if you were holding back urine, and then relax it for three seconds. Repeat ten times consecutively, three times a day.
- Increase contraction time (as the days go along) to fifteen seconds, up from three for each contraction. Repeat twenty-five times, four times a day.

...TO STRENGTHEN THE VAGINA:

- Contract the PC muscle for three seconds and release it for another three seconds. Repeat this action ten times consecutively and do it three times a day.
- Increase the duration of the contractions and relaxations up to fifteen seconds each. Also, increase the number of practice periods per day, though it is not advisable to exceed four.

"ORAL" ORGASMS

Both sexes usually agree that orgasms obtained by oral sex are neither better nor worse than those obtained from intercourse, just different. Depending on their skill using tongue or lips, the result can be very deep orgasms, even more than with classic penetration. The warmth of the breath over very sensitive erogenous areas, the moisture of the tongue and saliva, and the added effect of a "submissive" posture are some of the components that can intensify an orgasm produced by oral sex.

Keep in mind that oral stimulation of your lady requires a lot more time than does yours. It's important to maintain a consistent rhythm of stimulation with your tongue around and on the clitoris. The majority of women require a substantial time (between fifteen and twenty minutes) of oral stimulation to reach orgasm. Some cannot reach climax by means of oral sex unless it is accompanied by penetration. For this reason, it is best to wait for the right time to perform oral sex on your partner, so that it doesn't become uncomfortable, or even annoying.

THE BENEFITS OF ORGASM

Besides being pleasurable, the latest research has demonstrated that orgasm affords numerous benefits on the psychological, as well as physical, level.

- **For starters, it burns fat.** Pelvic movements, increased heart rate, and dilation of the blood vessels of the genitals involved in foreplay and orgasm all expend energy. Though the amount burned varies—depending on what positions are employed, how long the session lasts, and the vigor of the movements—it is possible to say that having sex including orgasm burns around 150 calories.

- **It has been confirmed** that when sexually excited, women produce large quantities of estrogen, the female sex hormone that supports smooth skin and shiny hair.

- **Estrogen stimulates circulation** and helps to protect women from heart disease. When a woman's body produces estrogen, her risk of heart attack is much less than that of a man.

- **Tranquilizer and analgesic.** Both are results of orgasm. Orgasm is ten times more effective than valium in relieving migraine headaches by lessening the tension of cerebral blood vessels, as well as reducing other pains.

- **During sexual foreplay** the secretion of oxytocin is increased, which promotes the experience of deep and powerful feelings. During orgasm, endorphins are released, causing sensations of well-being; prolactin, which is an anti-stress hormone, is also liberated, as well as serotonin, which gives rise to feelings of total happiness.

- The increase in levels of these hormones in a woman also **reduces the risk of maladies of the vaginal tract.** In addition, they delay the onset of osteoporosis, relieve symptoms of arthritis and menstruation, and protect against hypertension.

- The National Cancer Institute of the United States, for its part, has published that orgasms **can reduce the risk of prostate cancer** up to one-third.

- **Having sex,** in whatever way, has been demonstrated to be a crucial factor in staying young. According to a study conducted by the investigator David Weeks of the Royal Edinburgh Hospital in Scotland, to have sex at least three times per week lengthens one's lifespan an average of ten years.
- **Besides giving pleasure,** orgasm and the sexual excitement which precedes it improve respiration and blood circulation. If practiced frequently, this can even result in increased levels of hemoglobin, a natural antibody which helps fight infection.

SOMEONE WRITES US...

That night it so happened that I went out with a few friends. I had been divorced for four months, and they persuaded me to go out to dinner and have a couple of drinks afterwards. At first, I didn't feel much like doing it, but I forced myself to forget my troubles, at least for one night. Dinner was very pleasant and afterwards we went to have a drink at a club that was opening that very night. There we met with my friends' son, a young man of twenty-five, architectural student and basketball player on the university team.

We began to chat and pretty soon we were sharing all of our troubles. My friends were really tired and soon left for home. I felt good and stayed a bit longer with Marcos (the good-looking architect).

We didn't stop dancing till 4 in the a.m., when he offered to take me home. I didn't want it to end there, and so I invited him in to have "one for the road." Things happened so fast. Sitting on my living-room sofa, he started kissing me all over my body. It had been a while since anyone had done that to me. I shyly took off my clothes and his tongue was all over me. He nibbled my neck, and licked my nipples, as his fingers made their way between my legs.

His tongue went down to my belly, where he played around a bit with my belly button, then he plunged his face into my sex. His warm breath and experienced tongue caused me to have my first orgasm of the night, and the first I'd ever had from oral stimulation. My husband had never been competent in this and, in fact, was squeamish about it. Believe me, I felt chills all over from top to bottom.

After several more orgasms, we fell asleep, exhausted, in the middle of a totally upended apartment. I never saw Marcos again. Getting involved with the son of my friends was not a good idea. But I treasure that night in my memory and, since then, I always rate my lovers according to the size of their tongue....

Teresa, 47 years old

Just About Her

We now arrive at the little "treasure house" of pleasure. It is where the most intense thrills are generated, the erogenous zone par excellence which, by mistake, clumsiness, or excessive vigor, many men engage in an out-of-control way, without any forethought.

Male sexual response is more rapid than the woman's. His capacity to become aroused, have an erection, and ejaculate can often seem to rival the *Guinness Book* record, much to the disappointment of his lover.

Pay special attention to the first part of this book. It talks about the importance of foreplay: caresses, kisses, surroundings, and everything else that revolves around this magic moment of preliminaries. Without them, the sexual act becomes something mechanical, predictable, and even worse, of little pleasure for either of the partners.

Did someone mention haste? Many men underestimate the time it takes for foreplay. The kisses, strokes, little licks, and nibbles are the best preamble to sex for any woman. (If you, the reader, are a female, have your lover/partner carefully read this chapter, starting here.) Normally, most men opt to "go for the gusto," concentrating on her nipples and genitals right from the start.

This rush to the destination, full speed ahead, deprives both of the pleasure of the journey. Coitus should never become the sole objective of lovemaking.

Generally, a good orgasm (one that gives you chills remembering it hours later) is reached when each and every one of the erogenous zones, beyond clitoris and nipples alone, have been adequately pleasured. Only in that way will the necessary level of excitement be reached and genital contact be welcome. It's the same thing as knocking at the door before entering, instead of just bursting in, unannounced. If your lover is one of those in a hurry, invite him to read the chapter on the erogenous zones and remind him that communication is the best friend of an excellent sexual relationship. Teach him how you like to be kissed and caressed. The idea is to explore each erotic zone so that he can discover what you enjoy the most.

THE FEMALE BODY REVEALED

Mount of Venus. This is a suggestive name used to refer to this section of soft tissue located on the pelvis and usually covered with hair. It protects the inner genitals and dampens the contact of coitus. Crisscrossed with numerous nerve endings, it is, along with the clitoris (which is located at the bottom of the Mount), one of the principal erogenous zones of a woman. To caress the pubic hair, to lick the area gently, or massage it delicately will prove to be a source of inexhaustible pleasure for her.

Removing the hair from here makes for greater sensitivity. It's been quite a while since shaving the pubic area has been considered taboo. In fact, after the armpits (75 percent) and the legs (80 percent), the crotch is the third most depilated and groomed area of women's bodies. Also, for couples who regularly practice oral sex, a pubic area which is trimmed and well-tended is something pleasant to encounter. To totally enjoy oral sex, it is important to maintain proper genital hygiene. Cleanly shaved pubic hair, at the very least, reduces the presence of unpleasant odors.

When it comes time to depilate or shape the "Mount of Venus," you need only imagination and fantasy. Many women opt for original colors and shapes for the "garland" of their pubis. A strawberry formed of pubic hairs dyed red, the silhouette of a drop of water or tear, the initials of a partner's name, and even the logo of one's company or business, one's favorite sports team, and trademarks, are the most sought-after motifs. Any of these can be done in special hairdressing establishments.

These are the four most popular styles:

- **Short Cut.** This consists in cutting the pubes short for comfort, hygiene, and esthetics.
- **Contour Cut.** A really close shave. Undies are getting skimpier, and we must adapt!
- **Brazilian.** This is a complete removal of hair, very popular in erotic films.
- **Shapes.** One can employ any myriad of geometric shapes.

Before beginning pubic or genital depilation (either male or female), you must keep in mind that this is a very sensitive area, unaccustomed to razor irritation. If you wish to avoid the nuisances associated with "intimate depilation," it is best to remove the hair gradually.

To start, remove some hair every day, over the course of a week, with a pair of small, sharp scissors. The idea is that the skin of the area will become used to the shearing and not become irritated. If you notice any stinging or chaffing, stop cutting and wait until the annoyance subsides.

When you decide to go ahead with a pubic shave, first give the area a good shower with warm water. This way you will soften the hair and facilitate cutting it with the razor. Speaking of razors, always choose models with a swiveling head and use a new one each time that you shave yourself. Do it at night or when you don't intend to leave home. This way you can dress yourself in something baggy and comfortable and avoid your clothes rubbing the area for several hours.

To depilate the pubis, apply abundant shaving cream and pull the skin with one hand, as you shave with the other. Take your time on the first pass, slowly going in the direction of the hairs (usually downwards).

Before you return for a second pass with the razor over the area not completely shaved, apply more shaving cream. Once you've finished, apply lotion or cream.

If you prefer to go to a salon which specializes in this type of hair removal, the most common depilation techniques for this most intimate area are:

- **Traditional Method.** Done with hair-removal wax at low temperature. This is the most sought-after method.
- **Sugar and Lemon Amalgam.** This is done using an ancient Egyptian technique that doesn't cause nicks or bruising. It is best for sensitive skins.
- **Laser.** This method is used when one wishes to avoid the possibility of nicking sensitive mucosal tissue with a razor. Its advantage is longer-lasting depilation compared to the above-mentioned methods and, to a large extent, the pubic hairs do not re-grow. It is recommended for deep depilation or for decorative depilation where precision is required. It is the most expensive of the methods.

Clitoral Hood. The clitoral hood corresponds to the foreskin of the penis of a man and is formed by the joining of the *labia majora* and *labia minora* of the vulva. Its function is to protect the glans and shaft of the clitoris. It is arrayed with sebaceous glands which make it shiny and allow it to easily slide over the glans, so as to allow constant stimulation without irritation during coitus.

This organ varies in size among women and is one of the most erogenous and pleasure-inducing zones available to a session of oral sex. The act of licking the hood, and withdrawing it gently to stimulate the clitoral glans, is usually extremely exciting for the majority of women. The best way to do this is to separate the lips, or lift the mons pubic.

Outer Lips. The outer or "big" lips are two fleshy folds which cover and protect the most delicate parts of the vulva. The outer face is covered with hair and the inner side is shiny. During sex, the lips swell and become red, due to the concentration of blood in this area.

Inner Lips. The inner or "little" lips are also two fleshy folds situated within the outer lips. They surround the clitoris and vaginal opening. They join at the top of the vulva and form the prepuce or hood of the clitoris.

The inner lips are extremely sensitive and vary in size and shape for each woman, so much so that it can be said the *labia minora* are as personal as a woman's fingerprints.

Being formed of spongy, erectile tissue, the little lips become excited and swell during the sex act. The structures of the little lips change greatly throughout the phases, from excitation to restoration; above all, they change in size and color. They are not excessively sensitive, but their elasticity allows the inner parts of the clitoris to expand outwards when they are filled with blood.

Clitoris: That Great Unknown. Up to this point in time, it seems impossible, but many men still do not know the anatomy, function, and way to stimulate this little button of feminine pleasure. It is a hooded structure, formed of erectile tissue, which acts like a big sponge and fills with blood when it is excited. It this regard, it acts just like the penis and grows in size. Stimulated, the visible part of the clitoris grows to three times its normal size. Its normal length is approximately one quarter-inch (7.5 mm), but most of it is hidden within the body. The most visible part is a rosy *glans*, small and smooth, and covered with a hood of skin.

The clitoris contains six thousand to eight thousand nerve endings, the same number as in the penis, charged with producing sexual pleasure in a woman. As such, we are talking about an area of high sensitivity and a structure with the greatest concentration of nerve endings in the body. It is joined to the *labia minora* of the vulva and is partially covered by them. In fact, only the prepuce and glans of the clitoris are visible, being found at the top part of the little lips, and which form scarcely a tenth of its size.

The visible part of the clitoris begins at a point where the big lips join, at the base of the Mount of Venus, and continues into a protuberance named the glans. The surface of the glans is covered with a hood whose function is to protect it from over-stimulation and irritation. For its part, the hood is joined with the glans underneath the skin.

The term "clitoris" comes from the Greek "kleitoris," which means "little mountain," and it is the only organ whose sole function is to provide sexual pleasure, pleasure which is the result of either manual or oral stimulation, as well as penetration. Let's take a moment to consider this point. For many women, stimulation of the clitoris by means of penetration alone proves to be insufficient. According to studies conducted by Shere Hite (Hite Report on Female Sexuality), 30 percent of women who have orgasms during coitus have them due to direct or indirect stimulation of the clitoris, and not to penetration alone.

In other words, every woman is different and has her own needs for stimulation of the clitoris. So, while some prefer firm pressure, there are others who melt with pleasure from the simplest of rubs, or rapid tapping. Some get excited when their lover licks or sucks their clitoris, while there are others who go wild when the penis presses it. In addition, there are different reactions of the clitoris after orgasm. With some women, it is necessary to wait a while before being able to touch it again. With others, you can start right away to stimulate it for a new climax, even several more times. In this case, it can happen that the sensations become even more intense with each succeeding orgasm.

Vaginal Opening. Located under the urethral opening, it is the beginning of a cylindrical tube, namely the vagina, which extends from the vulva to the neck of the womb.

The vagina's walls are muscular and covered with a mucosal lining, being very elastic and readily lubricated. The most erogenous areas are situated near the vaginal opening. Due to its inherent pliability (it can open and close, allow entry or stop it, depending on the level of its excitation), oral sex is very pleasurable in this area. Stimulating the perineum while engaging in oral sex is extremely enjoyable.

The Perineum. Not far from the clitoris and pubic mound is one of the most erotogenic areas of the female genitals. It is a strip of muscular tissue situated between the vulva and anus. Its principal function is to support the organs housed in the pelvic cavity.

Though less sensitive than the clitoris, this area near the anus proves to be very erotic in some women, responding very readily to finger pressure or circular strokes. With oral stimulation, it is very pleasurable to run the tip of the tongue over the perineum while gently pressing the muscle with fingers. If your lover rests his hand over this area with the external lips of the vagina closed, and presses it vigorously or massages it, he can quickly excite you, due to the dense network of nerve endings which are gathered there.

The big secret of oral sex on a woman, cunnilingus, is tenderness, a delicate touch, and rhythm. We've already noted that women need foreplay, those preliminaries which little by little wake up desire and excitement. Female sexual response is slower than a male's. And therein lies the big mistake of men. It's just the way they think; they go full speed ahead, even sometimes roughly, turning oral sex into a clumsy and rushed affair. Again we insist: have your guy read the earlier chapters that deal with foreplay; the kisses, caresses, sensual massage, etc.

THE ART OF KISSING

Lips are extremely sensitive and erogenous, so much so that a good kissing session is the best way to "get her motor started." It's advisable to start sensuously, slowly, with lips half-open. Press them lightly against those of your lover (they will fit together better if you put either your partner's upper or lower lip between yours). Kiss long, sweetly, savoring the moment. Little by little, separate your lips and let the point of your tongue begin to gently explore inside your lover's mouth. Wait until both tongues meet, then let them entwine. Withdraw your tongue slowly and lick your partner's lower lip, softly.

It's usually just about now that his hands go straight for the breasts or, even worse, the genitals. What's the rush? We're just getting started, so don't spoil it with your uncontrolled nervousness!

Take time to affectionately stroke her hair, her face, and her skin. Whisper to her how much you want her, how she excites you, and how you are going to make her melt with pleasure. Let your imagination go; show her she is about to experience intense sensations she's never had before.

Go down her neck, kissing, licking, and nibbling it softly. And don't be ashamed when it comes time to ask her what she likes, what she wants; just don't make a big deal about it. And don't forget that you have a fantastic pair of hands and arms. Kisses paired with hugs and gentle strokes are much more exciting and seductive.

Now it's time to go down the sides of her neck (be careful not to tickle her) and start stimulating her breasts. Do this without abrupt movements, with all the delicacy and care you muster. You are not kneading bread. Forget about pinches and nibbling here. The breasts are very sensitive; your warm breath alone can excite them. Cover the breasts with light kisses and licks, but don't touch the nipples yet. Move your tongue in spirals, moving closer to the nipples with each successive pass.

To stimulate the female breasts, you can choose among the following techniques:

- **Hot Breath.** Before touching her nipples, blow on them with your hot breath, but don't even brush against them.
- **The Whirlpool.** Move the tip of your tongue around the areola of her nipple, like a whirlpool, moving closer and closer to its tip. Start very slowly, increasing the rate of the swirls as you go along.
- **Trembling Tongue.** Vibrate your tongue back and forth over her nipple. Start slowly, and then pick up the pace.
- **Suction.** Gently, bring the nipple to your open mouth. Suck it; rub it with your tongue and lips. Squeeze it between your tongue and palate.
- **Suction and Whirlpool.** Using suction to hold the nipple inside your mouth, move your tongue around the nipple in a swirling motion. Start slowly and increase the speed as you go along.
- **Nibbling.** Nibble her nipple very gently. Don't do this for too long; the nipples are super delicate.
- **Simply Edible.** Take the nipple into your mouth, as far as you can, including as much of the breast as possible. Tenderly

rub your tongue all around, pressing the nipple and breast against your palate.

- **A Fresh Breath.** Finish by blowing on her moist nipples, giving them a pleasant, cool sensation. You can also use an ice cube held between your lips, running over her nipples as you softly massage the sides of her back.

CUNNILINGUS: ONWARD TO THE GRAND TREASURE!

At this point, your lady's level of excitement will be very high. But don't let yourself get carried away, not yet anyway. Go downwards slowly, covering her entire abdomen with kisses and caresses.

Next stop: the navel. Play with it; put your tongue inside, but just be careful not to tickle her; this is a very sensitive zone. At this point, you have two choices. You can go down to her thighs (don't even think about touching her genitals), or ask her to turn over so you can stimulate one of the body's most forgotten areas during sex: the back. Go over her spinal column from top to bottom with your fingertips, tongue, and lips, eventually reaching her butt (for many women one of the most erotic areas of their body). You can even be a little bit rough with her here with your massages and sucking (just be sure not to be too rough).

Forget her anus, for the moment. Leave it for later. Run your tongue along the crack of her butt while you softly massage her inner thighs. Let your warm breath approach her vagina, but don't touch her there yet.

Another erogenous zone that is relatively unknown is the backside of the knees. Run your tongue over them (this can cause considerable tickling) and then go down to her feet. Ask her or gently motion for her to turn over, face up.

Open her thighs and use your thumbs to separate the big lips of her vagina. Remember, the key to providing maximum excitation with cunnilingus is to make sure the clitoris and vulva are sufficiently lubricated before you start to stimulate them. Moisten your tongue and lips with saliva (you can also dab some on her sensitive area) and start kissing and sucking the lips of her vagina. Go over them with your tongue; lick them and play with them.

When this area is sufficiently lubricated and excited, begin to caress her clitoris with the end of your tongue (many men jump right on the clitoris without thought or previous preparation: a big mistake!). Press the glans with the tip of your tongue and use the tongue to go around it.

If you want to really boost the stimulation, try raising your girl's legs (grasp her thighs and move her legs so they rest on your shoulders). Next, softly lick her vulva and then press up on her rump so you can sink your tongue into her vagina. In this position, the man can deeply stimulate his partner's clitoris.

The key to successful cunnilingus is to start slowly, gently stimulating the area, and increasing the rhythm little by little. Each series of movements/stimulation should last about ten seconds: five seconds of licking a specific area, and then five seconds over the whole vagina itself. Use your fingers to elevate the Mount of Venus with each lick (this way the vestibule of the vagina will contract and the lips will move closer together) and release it when your tongue rests on the vulva.

Breathe all over her vulva and begin to caress the outer lips with the point of your tongue. Make long passes, soft and sustained. Remember you must start slowly and only then gradually increase your rhythm. Bit by bit, move your tongue closer to the clitoris, softly licking her little lips. Keeping your mouth slightly open on her vulva, make little circles around the clitoris with your tongue.

With your fingers, retract the hood of the clitoris (only if it's sufficiently aroused) so you can stimulate it directly. You are in the most sensitive area, so be very careful with your movements and use only the tip of your tongue to stimulate it. You can even stop a while, letting her continue her rhythmic movements, and find the points that cause her the most excitement when they are stimulated.

Cunnilingus is not limited to using the tongue alone. Sink your face between her legs, exhale your breath on her, and hide your nose in her Venus Mount. Then rest your upper lip and mustache area on the edge of her sacrum.

Continue moving the point of your tongue back and forth over your lover's clit. Start slowly, and gradually pick up the pace until you arrive at the velocity which excites her most.

Let her clitoris rest a bit, and introduce your tongue into her vagina. This is about penetrating as deeply as you can and keeping your mouth in constant contact with her. Go back to stimulating her clitoris, but this time suck it and rub it with tongue, lips, and mouth.

Don't forget to use your hands and fingers. During cunnilingus you can also softly massage her butt, rub her inner thighs, stimulate her perineum and anus, etc.

And now the great, golden rule: keep up rhythmic stimulation, without stopping, until she explodes in pleasure. You'll know she's about to orgasm when her body tenses. This is the way to make sure she keeps on the road to climax!

THE BEST TECHNIQUES

Can you move your tongue in circles? Good. Can you move it up and down and sideways? Perfect. Can you speed up and slow down the rhythm? Incredible! Could you draw a "figure eight" with your tongue tip? If you can perform all these movements, your partner is in luck because you are ready for the following techniques:

• **Naughty Circles.** Drawing circles with the point of your tongue is one of the most common, but exciting techniques for her. It's better not to press too hard, since the clitoris is sensitive and you don't want to injure it. Make spirals

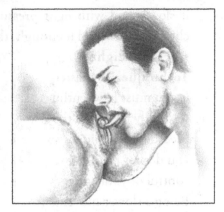

starting outside and work inward. You can make them small, medium, or large, clockwise or counterclockwise.

• **Vertical.** A movement which is very simple and gives her great pleasure is the vertical (upwards and downwards). Though it's easy to do, the biggest danger is that the man will speed up and do it too fast and with too much force. Do it with a flat tongue, and relaxed.

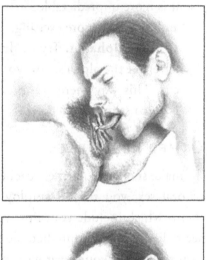

• **Side to Side.** Though this is the most difficult movement, it is the most pleasure-giving. The difficulty lies in avoiding a "superficial" cunnilingus; therefore, the tongue should caress and gently separate the lips. First, do

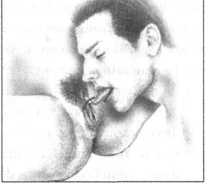

it slowly and with light pressure. Once you have located the clitoris and excited it enough, then increase speed and pressure.

- **Figure Eight Technique.** To master it you must have enthusiastically practiced the preceding techniques so you do not readily lose control of your tongue. Being a slower movement than the "naughty circle" and being more sinuous, it is more unpredictable and therefore more exciting.

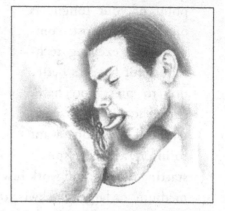

- **Sexy Alphabet.** Try to draw the letters of the alphabet on your girl's clit. This way there are a lot more ways to stimulate her!

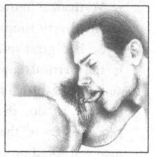

OTHER RESOURCES

To make sure your partner reaches climax with an exciting session of oral sex, you should employ various combinations of movements which include your lips, your tongue, and mouth, etc. The secret lies in being unpredictable and taking advantage of each session to surprise your lover with new moves and approaches. Here, follow some ideas to complete your tongue's training:

- **Humming.** Humming consists of making small, guttural sounds with your tongue on her sexual part. The vibrations generated this way act as an exciting mini-vibrator, which will drive your partner crazy.
- **Use Your Fingers.** Fingers are your best friends when doing cunnilingus. Introduce a finger into the vaginal

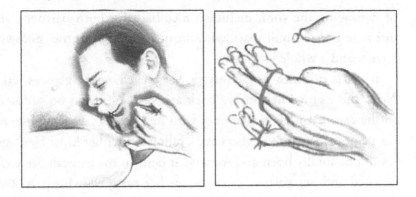

opening as you stimulate her clitoris with your tongue. Move your tongue softly, using it like a penis—entering, withdrawing, and twisting it. This combination of oral and manual sex is very exciting to a woman.

- **Lips and Teeth.** These are excellent complements to the tongue. For example, the lips can be used to surround the clitoris while the tongue pushes it up and down. Lips and tongue also help to uncover the clitoris when it is hidden behind the folds of the vulva.

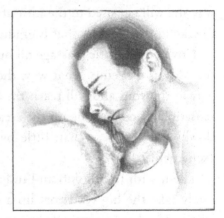

MASSAGING THE "YONI"

"Yoni" is the Sanskrit name for the vagina and means "sacred temple." Massaging the yoni is one of the most pleasurable tantric practices available to a woman.

In Tantra, most sexual activities are performed as rituals and, as with any ritual, require certain preparations which, in the case of massaging the yoni, include a nice bath for both partners, an intimate and tranquil space with music, candles, incense, pillows, scents, and a whole lot of time.

It starts off with hugs, soft caresses, exchanging glances, etc. Next, the woman lies on her back and rests her head on pillows, so she can maintain eye contact with her lover as well as observe the genitals. She should also have a pillow under her hips. Her legs should be totally open and somewhat bent so the genitals are well exposed and her partner can massage her easily. For his part, the man should sit between the woman's legs with his legs crossed, or in the "lotus" position.

It is important not to begin with direct massage of the yoni. First caress other parts of her body such as her legs, her crotch, breasts, stomach, and little by little close in on the "Sacred Temple." This way she will get used to the idea of being stroked and will be able to take in the pleasure that is gradually increasing.

Now, pour a little massage oil on your hands and gently stroke the Mount of Venus. That way, the oil will cover all of the outer part of the yoni and will reach the big lips, boosting the woman's sensations and warming up the area. The massage should be done slowly and gently so that, little by little, she experiences greater excitement.

Then, with the thumb and index finger, the man should delicately take the big (exterior) lip and squeeze it, sliding along its length. He should gently do the same with the little lips.

Now use circular strokes around the clitoris, going clockwise, and then counter-clockwise. Softly press the clitoris directly, using the thumb and index finger.

Continuing, and with great care, introduce the middle finger of the right hand into the yoni. Using the right hand is important, since this way you maintain the correct energetic polarity as indicated by the Tantra. Explore the interior of the yoni with your finger, changing speeds, pressure, and direction. Move further inward, as if to put your hand in up to its palm, and stimulate your partner's "G" spot.

You can also introduce your ring finger and continue massaging, while the thumb gently stimulates the clitoris.

By now, she should be at a high level of excitation. You can keep going until she reaches climax, or wait a few moments and then return to gently continue stimulation of the area.

Just About Him

Many say the penis is a man's only erogenous zone. It's true that his sexual response is very quick, and generally, sexual excitation is confined, almost exclusively, to this area. But men, too, enjoy foreplay. Kisses, stroking, massages, licks, whispers—all are necessary for a man's full enjoyment, if it is to be more than just simple coitus. The same skill, tenderness, and patience are required from you to make him come undone with pleasure.

Caresses are not the exclusive prerogative of women. Men also like it when you run your delicate little hands over their body and massage those erogenous zones (it's true, they *do* have them) in a seductive, naughty way.

For example, you might start with a relaxing head massage. If you have long nails, take advantage of them and make gentle circles all over his scalp. Get naked and place his head on your knees. With your hands extended on both sides of his head, behind his ears, exert light pressure with your fingers, keeping them slightly bent. Place your fingertips in his hair and massage it, as if you were giving him a shampoo, but always with slow movements and applying light pressure. With circular movements, move your fingers back and forth, going down to the nape of his neck and pressing his forehead with your thumbs.

This area of the skin is very susceptible to caressing, but don't go too far with it, since that will cause him to relax to the point of sleepiness. And that is not what you want at this moment.

Keeping the same position, you can now go down to his neck, and then his chest, even massaging his nipples with your fingers. A man's nipples are exceedingly sensitive to stroking, kissing, and even soft pinching (take it between your thumb and index finger).

You can also play with the hair on his chest, stroking it, tugging it gently, taking it in your lips, etc.

Indeed, the key with men is the same as with you: start slowly and gradually build up the level of stimulation. Remember, *you* are in control. You do not want to go too fast and trigger his already rapid and direct sexual response. The secret is to always begin by stimulating with foreplay. This way, you stretch things out until he's ready for a massage.

Have him lie face down and begin with a gentle massage all over his back. Run your fingertips over his skin until you sense it bristling with pleasure. You can use the palms of your hands as well as your fingers, sliding them softly, without any haste. Work on his neck first, moving down to the shoulders, arms, back, legs, and all the way down to his feet.

Then go back the way you came, passing over the same areas as you return to his neck. You can use your hands for this massage, but don't forget you have lips, a tongue, and even your breasts as alternatives.

If you want to add a more erotic touch, warm a bit of massage oil in your hands and rub it on your partner's back. Use soft, sliding strokes along its length, following the path of his spine. Place your open hands on it with your fingers parallel, sliding downwards with light pressure. Then go upwards, this time exerting pressure with just the base of your hand.

Men receive pleasure from deep and energetic massage. For this, you can use kneading as a technique. This consists of taking hold of the muscle in your hand and plying it, using your thumb and the rest of your fingers in opposition. Start with the shoulders and descend, bit by bit, to his back.

By now, your boy is ready for more seductive stimulation. Massage his butt and the inside of his thighs, slowly approaching his genitals.

CENTER OF HIS UNIVERSE

The penis—that small, yet great volcano—is the erotic zone par excellence of men, the place concentrating their most intense and pleasurable sensations. The whole penis is very sensitive, but its end, the glans, is particularly rich in nerve endings and above all the corona of the glans, which responds extremely rapidly to minimal stimulation. The frenum of the foreskin is also a place of extreme sensitivity, as well as just behind the opening of the penis.

Let's get to know them a little better.

Scrotum and Testicles. The scrotum is the external sack which holds the testicles. It is of two unequal parts, with the left side usually descending lower than the right. Both testicles are incredibly sensitive to erotic stimulation.

The scrotum is analogous to the outer lips of the vagina, and though caresses and kisses do cause deep sensations, it is best to stimulate it delicately, since it is such a delicate organ. If you spread a bit of massage oil on the scrotum, that will help to manipulate it more smoothly and avoid any painful tugging.

Glans, Prepuce, and Frenum. The penis is formed of three spongy cylinders which, when excited, fill with blood and make it erect. At the end of the penis there exists a protuberance, the glans, usually covered with a piece of skin (the foreskin).

Both the glans and foreskin are full of nerve endings, and stimulating them causes great pleasure. The glans and foreskin are joined on the underside of the penis by a piece of skin named the frenum, or "V" point. This is the most excitable part of the penis and, stimulated by itself, can result in orgasm. It's preferable not to begin stimulation with this part, but to approach it gradually after having explored other areas. Be careful: stimulate the "V" spot with great gentleness; the slightest contact is enough to inundate it with sensation.

The glans is very susceptible to caressing with the lips, tongue, saliva, or teeth (delicately—it is quite fragile). Focus your most sensual caresses on this part. You can, for example, hold the penis firmly upright and make little circles on the glans, polishing it from one side to the other and up and down. You can also put your fingertips over the head of the glans, as if covering it over with a closed umbrella, and squeeze upwards towards the outside of its end. Also stimulate the groove of the glans with the point of your tongue or end of your thumb, always being very careful and making sure to watch your guy's reactions.

Due to the extreme sensitivity of these areas of the penis, most of the stimulation should be done orally, since contact with the tongue tends to be much softer than that of the hands or fingers. You can give little flicks of the tongue or gentle licks, making circles on it, alternating with vertical and horizontal passes.

In case you use your fingers or some other part of your body or some object, make sure the area is well lubricated to ensure smooth contact.

Crest of the Corona. This is the posterior part of the glans which sticks out. It is very sensitive, and you can stimulate it by circling your tongue around it and licking it underneath. Another seductive stroke consists of taking the skin at the base of the penis, forming a ring around it with your thumb and forefinger, and turning them around the penis at just the point where the glans begins.

Stem. This is the main part of the penis and is most sensitive at its back. Grasp it firmly (without overdoing it) and make back and forth movements. You can combine this with a good session of oral sex.

Perineum. Situated between the scrotum and anus, this zone is very sensitive, as much in men as in women. In fact, it's even more sensitive in men due to the presence of the prostate just under the skin.

Use your tongue to stimulate here, gently passing over the area, or caressing it with your fingertips, as well as kissing it, or delicately massaging. You can also press firmly with one or two fingers right behind the scrotum. Don't do this for more than a second, though. If you want, you can repeat this motion a few times. Remember that stimulating the perineum combined with oral sex makes for something extremely pleasurable.

The prostate gland may be stimulated by direct pressure on the perineum. Consisting of the external wall of the prostate, the perineum has been compared to the famous "G" spot in women.

A QUESTION OF **SIZE**

- Small Penis*..... Less than 4" (12 cm)......3% of men
- Medium Penis*.....Between 4" and 6" (12 cm and 17 cm)......79% of men
- Large Penis*.....Over 6" (17 cm)......18% of men
  The diameter is usually between 1" and 1" (3 cm and 4.2 cm).

*Measured when erect

MASSAGING THE "LINGAM"

"Lingam" is the Sanskrit word which refers to the male sexual organ. You're about to learn a Tantric massage for this area, which will drive your guy nuts with pleasure.

First have him lie down, face up, with several pillows under his head (so that the head and torso are raised). He should be comfortable, with his knees slightly bent and legs apart. In this position his genitals should be completely exposed for the massage to be totally effective.

Warm a little massage oil in your hands and spread it on his penis (or lingam) and testicles. Start massaging his scrotum and testicles, making sure they are relaxed. Rub his perineum gently (between the testicles and anus) and continue with the lingam, changing pressure and speed so as to increase his pleasure.

With your right hand, press the base of his penis. Slide your hand up and down, alternating with your left hand as well. Continue these movements and then press the head of the lingam, alternating your hands.

Remember the aim of this Tantric massage is not to bring him to ejaculation. In every way, by now, your lover will be totally aroused, so back off a bit from further stimulation.

Now it's time to massage the "Sacred Point" (perineum). To do this, you can press the zone gently with your left hand while you continue to use your right hand to massage the lingam.

Continue this way for a few minutes, until he reaches orgasm.

FELLATIO: MAKE HIM MELT WITH PLEASURE!

To give your lover a gift of stimulating fellatio is pretty straightforward. The key is to enjoy giving it as much or more than the one receiving it. It is important to start with the preliminaries, which are totally worth the effort. Caresses, kisses, massage, scents, tastes—all are used so that excitation keeps mounting in intensity, even before your mouth so much as touches his penis. You have various methods at your disposal: you can gently rub your breasts on his genitals, go over his nipples with the point of your tongue, kiss his body from stem to stern. . . all with your imagination at the helm!

Try to not repeat movements or positions. Surprise him with different approaches and ideas. Sure, he has just one thing on his mind. But *you* are in control; calm any concerns he may have and go over his entire skin before you fellate him. Lick his neck, lick his nipples, lick his belly, play with his belly button, and warm up his genitals with your hot breath, without touching them.

The moment has come: take his penis at its base with one hand and, using the other, massage his butt, anus, legs, and scrotum. Free his glans from its hood and bring it to your moist lips.

Form an "O" with your lips, rest them on the tip of his penis, and move your head in small circles.

Now is the time to fix your lips on his shaft and go over it, from one side to the other. Grab the end of his penis between your lips; make rapid turns, kissing it and tugging backwards on its delicate skin. Let his glans slide all the way into your mouth and squeeze the shaft firmly between your two lips.

Everything you do should be aimed at getting him to really enjoy the experience. While holding his penis, move your hand up and down; open your hand slightly as you near the base and close it as you get close to the glans. As your hand goes down, position your head over his penis so you can take it deeper into your mouth. Keep his penis moving in and out of your mouth (with lips covering your teeth); use firm, but comfortable pressure. Lick his penis, going over its shaft and glans in particular. Nibble with your lips and use a lot of saliva; the better the lubrication, the better it will feel. Finally, put his penis in your mouth and run your tongue around his glans. Change directions as you move your tongue around; let your saliva cover it and press his frenum with both palate and tongue. Use your hands to massage his testicles, perineum, and anus.

Play with your partner by changing rhythms; move quickly, suck harder, and then slow down so he doesn't reach orgasm.

When you move away, you can hold his penis with just one hand, or else leave your lips resting on the tip of the glans, so you can resume sucking immediately. In either case, make sure your hand remains around his penis, the back of the hand facing your mouth.

Another basic, very exciting fellation technique consists of taking the shaft of the penis with your hand and twisting the skin as you stimulate the glans with your tongue, or, with your tongue-tip go over the corona of the glans and toy with his frenum.

Know that a man's sexual response to fellatio is going to be very quick. When you notice he's at his highest point of excitation, remove your lips from the penis and begin licking and nibbling his scrotum and testicles. You can also abate an imminent eruption by massaging his perineum for a few moments.

DIFFERENT FELLATIO TECHNIQUES

- Lick or suck the shaft of the penis; from back to front is the best way.
- Lick or suck the glans (careful, for many men this can be annoying or painful).
- Nibble or rub the glans (make sure it's well lubricated).
- Stroke, nibble, or lick his frenum and the ring of the glans.
- Press or stretch the frenum (be careful, as excessive force can cause irritation).

- Lick or gently nibble the scrotum, always from underneath to the top.
- Put your tongue in the gap of his glans.
- Any oral sex practice becomes much more exciting and pleasant when accompanied by manual stimulation (masturbation, pressure at the base of the penis, gentle fondling of the testicles, pressure on the ring of the scrotum, stroking the shaft of the penis, etc.).

USE YOUR IMAGINATION

- **BUTTERFLY WINGS.** Pass your tongue rapidly over his frenum and take his penis, holding more of it in your hand than your mouth, making sure to keep your teeth covered with your lips so as not to hurt the delicate skin of the glans.
- **TOTAL SUCTION.** With his penis in your mouth, close your lips around it and suck hard, pressing the penis against the palate with your tongue. Move your tongue over the frenum. If you prefer, take the penis halfway in your mouth and suck vigorously. You can also do this with the glans alone. When you notice your lover's breathing is speeding up or his movements indicate he is about to orgasm, back off, and lightly pull on his testicles.
- **DELICIOUS CHILLS.** Chill your mouth with an ice cube and then massage his frenum with your cold tongue.

DID YOU KNOW THAT...?

The word "fellatio" comes from the Latin "fellare," which means to suck.

The prostitutes of Phoenicia and ancient Egypt would paint their lips to advertise to their clients that they performed fellatio.

Cleopatra's enemies spread the rumor that she was a great expert of fellatio. They said she practiced fellatio on her soldiers to conserve her youthfulness and vitality, given the "magical" qualities of semen.

In the Roman Empire, those who practiced fellatio and cunnilingus were looked down upon, but not those who received it. The worst insult a Roman could get was if someone told him he had practiced fellatio on another man. Equally, the worst threat was to *force* someone to practice fellatio on another man.

SHOULD I SWALLOW HIS SEMEN?

This is a very personal decision. If you don't want his semen to enter your mouth, you must tell him beforehand so he takes his penis out of your mouth at the first spasms of ejaculation. It's important, however, that you don't stop suddenly right at the moment of climax: keep masturbating until he's done. Maybe you don't want his semen in your mouth, but a very exciting alternative is to let his semen spill on your breasts, neck, or face.

If you don't mind swallowing his semen, continue to suck lightly as you notice he is coming and keep on until his penis totally loses its hardness in your mouth.

Most important is to be sure your lover is not infected with any STDs. Ingestion of any bodily fluids or oral to genital contact carry with them the risk of contagion.

Whatever your preference, the most important thing is to end your oral sex session in a seductive and exciting way. It's important nothing causes disgust or repulsion, since this can ruin the magic of the moment.

It's understandable that you might not like the taste or texture of semen. A good alternative to keep the climax erotic, if you chose

> not to swallow, is to let his semen run over his penis so you can give him a final hot and wet massage. The idea is not to take ejaculation as something "dirty" or repulsive.

How Does Semen Taste?

We are what we eat. This goes for the taste of all our bodily fluids, including semen. This means, for example, if the diet is heavy in foods rich in sugars, the semen will taste sweet and pleasant. On the other hand, if he overdoes the proteins (meat, fish, etc.), the semen will have a more sour taste and odor. In general, the foods which give semen a better taste are fruits (especially plums, mangos, pineapple, and all kinds of citrus).

The texture, taste, odor, and quantity of semen ejaculated are different for each man. It is not a case of "one size fits all." Quantity (as well as texture) will vary depending on the size of the prostate and frequency of sexual relations.

As we've already said, the taste depends on what he eats and includes the effects of other substances such as tobacco or alcohol:

- **Bitter:** consumption of alcohol and tobacco.
- **Sour:** red meat, asparagus, cabbage, broccoli, spinach, coffee, and multi-vitamins.
- **Sweet:** rice, potatoes, pastries, and all types of carbohydrates.
- **Tasteless:** fresh vegetables.

In a recent Internet survey on the taste of semen, the responders voted as follows:

- I do not like the taste..........8.5%
- I like it.........................15.5%
- I never tried it....................52%

- It tastes sour......................9%
- It tastes bitter....................11%
- It tastes sweet....................4%

Semen is composed of various nutrients, including ascorbic acid, citric acid, creatine, magnesium, fructose, lactic acid, sodium, sorbitol, vitamin B_{12}, and zinc, among others.

The average volume of semen in an ejaculation varies between one-tenth fluid ounce to one-fifth fluid ounce (3 ml to 5 ml), with a maximum around one-half fluid ounce (one tablespoon, 15 ml). The amount varies according to frequency of sexual relations and the degree of sexual excitement of the man. The amount of semen produced increases with age to a maximum, which depends on the individual. After this, the amount produced decreases, although the individual will keep producing semen for the rest of his life.

Regarding oral sex, semen can be swallowed without any ill effects. It is not fattening, and will cause no harm, as long as the man doesn't suffer from any contagious diseases. The only thing to avoid is getting ejaculate in the eyes, as this can irritate the mucous membrane of the eye, producing temporary discomfort.

TASTES AND SMELLS

It's obvious that the practice of oral sex requires scrupulous hygiene of the genitals. Though there are people who are OK with their own smell, if you are going to have oral sex after a hard and long day at work, taking a shower together or enjoying a bubble bath would be a good way to start foreplay.

To thoroughly clean the penis, retract the foreskin carefully, wash the front and back of the glans as well as the frenum. Use ordinary bath gel and rinse abundantly with water. If you're still not 100 percent sure about your partner, have him use a condom before you fellate him. There are varieties in different flavors which can make the session more flavorful!

TRICKS OF THE TRADE

If you want to leave your lover breathless, here are some secrets for giving him the best fellatio of his life:

- Before you start, have something hot to drink. There is nothing more exciting to a man than to feel a hot tongue and palate running over his penis.
- Submission is one of the most exciting sexual fantasies. Let him dominate you; follow his commands, kneeling in front of him. Other guys prefer just the opposite; you can tie him up to the bedposts, blindfold him, and suck him till he loses his mind!
- Bondage consists of tying up your partner so that he can hardly move. It is a very kinky practice of domination. You can use silk handkerchiefs, ties, stockings, or similar items of clothing. The key is to make your slave suffer. The master must toy with the slave's excitation, doing what she knows will bring him to a place just short of total arousal, and then stop, leaving him begging for more. The man-slave will beg, more and more; his body will arch, he will plead, but it all depends on the one in control. To make it more kinky, she can even blindfold him.
- If you want your partner to go straight to climax, introduce a finger in his anus or use your thumb to apply pressure to his perineum.
- What excites them most is everything you do before your mouth ever touches their penis. Remember, the more you provoke their excitement, the more intense their orgasm will be.

- Continual sucking and tongue stimulation are vital. If you want to get him to orgasm, speed up the rhythm until his respiration rate increases, he's groaning more, his body starts to twitch involuntarily, etc.

- Pinching different spots on his body creates an incredible sensation of both pleasure and pain. Before you go looking for clothespins to do this, be aware there are special aids available in sex shops. You can apply these pincers on many parts of your lover's body like the nipples, the butt, big and little lips of the vulva, the penis, the clitoris, etc. Some advice: if you are new to this sort of thing it's better to start out on less sensitive places, like the butt.

- Waxing is a daring way to experience sex on that line between pleasure and pain. It consists of pouring hot wax, with utmost care, on your bodies. One of the two is the "master." The "slave" is tied up. The master alternates a couple of minutes of pouring wax with a couple of minutes of masturbation or oral sex: a combination of pain and pleasure.

In any event, with wax you must keep several things in mind. It is best to use paraffin wax, since it melts at a lower temperature than other waxes. The most manageable candles are two and a quarter inches in diameter (6 cm) and four and three quarter inches (12 cm) in length. Make a small notch at the edge of the candle so you can control pouring the wax on your lover's skin. With this, the best thing to do would be to pour the wax on open areas of skin or hair.

To do it seductively, hold the candle over a small stretch of skin and tilt it a little at a time. Remember that the closer you hold the candle to the skin, the more heat will be delivered. Keep a bowl of cold water nearby so you can throw some on in a hurry if the wax is too hot. And finally, to remove the wax, the best way is to rub over it with an ice cube and take it off with a plastic scrapper.

ERRORS TO AVOID

- **There is a technique for everything.** It's not just a simple matter of giving him fellatio and then he melts in pleasure. There are certain things which, if done, can bring down his desire during fellatio.
- **Biting prohibited.** All of a man's genitals, especially the glans and frenum, are sensitive. Make sure that when you give him fellatio you have your teeth covered over with your lips at all times.
- **Enjoy it yourself.** 50 percent of the success of good fellatio depends on the involvement and enjoyment of the one giving it. There are women who practice oral sex automatically, as if someone else were doing it. Resolve to show him, in every moment, how much you enjoy giving him pleasure. Don't skimp on murmurs, sighs, or little grunts. Practice humming, which is nothing but the sound generated in your throat with the intent to provoke a pleasant, tingling sensation in the genital area of the person receiving oral sex.
- **Don't be too rough.** Avoid pulling the foreskin too hard, or gripping the penis too tightly, as if trying to uproot it. Remember, saliva is the best aid to good fellatio. Besides being a lot more exciting, it will help you make more smooth and fluid movements.
- **Semen is not poisonous.** It's up to you whether to swallow or not; just don't wretch when the first drop of semen shows up, and don't run off to the bathroom to gargle if some gets in your mouth.

- **The most important thing of all** is to "listen" to your partner's body, to be aware of what he likes or if he wants you to go faster or slower, or if he wants you to change the rhythm.

GET COMFORTABLE

There's a certain tempo required for good fellatio, as well as a comfortable position for both partners which allows easy access to the man's genitals. In addition, when the penis is erect, it works best that whoever is giving fellatio has their face perpendicular to the man's penis. Men are very susceptible to visual stimuli; therefore, a position which allows him to see you unhindered is advisable.

The usual position is for the man to lie back, face up, with his head slightly raised so he doesn't miss any of the "show." This way, the one giving fellatio has access to all parts of his penis and testicles. It is a position which allows the best angle for the penis to easily enter the mouth and is very comfortable for the man.

Another way is to have the man on his knees or standing. This can be uncomfortable for the one giving fellatio, but it leaves the giver completely free to use her hands to massage her partner. This is a really great way to do "the butterfly stroke." This is a fellatio technique that is very stimulating and consists of lightly running the tongue along the length of the frenum or underneath the penis. The man can stroke his partner's hair while this is going on, but he must be careful not to push or move her head, since this can cause her to gag.

A very interesting position is the one where the person giving fellatio stretches comfortably on the bed, facing up, with the head slightly elevated (you can put a cushion underneath). The man strides up to her on his knees so that his penis is at the same level as her mouth. She then has total access to the penis and testicles and can also stimulate the anus, perineum, as well as his crotch, using her hands. She can also indulge in some "self-stimulation" to boot. The man will be able to caress his partner's body, this being a position which is very comfortable for both.

Oral Kama Sutra

Don't be a boring lover. The golden rule of sex is to bring some imagination and fantasy to your sexual encounters. There is nothing more exciting than to surprise (or be surprised) with new positions, different places, new adventures. . . in short, to find that "kinky little something extra" that sets our desire on fire.

So, open up all your senses and get yourself ready to dive into the ancient text of the *Kama Sutra*. One can translate this title from the Sanskrit as "The Way of Love." "Kama" means physical passion/desire (it is also the name of the minor Hindu god in charge of these matters) and "sutra" means "aphorism," or the expression of an idea in the fewest words possible. This manual, compiled in the fourth century A.D. by the erudite Hindu Vatsyayana, encourages uninhibited exploration of sexual positions and techniques. The author presents sex as a human need, which we should not repress, but rather cultivate and enjoy. According to this book, the union of two people is both physically and spiritually significant. Eros is both necessary and advisable, but happiness, not orgasm, is the ultimate aim.

It wasn't until 1883 that the *Kama Sutra* arrived in Europe by way of an English edition produced by Richard Burton and

F. F. Arbuthnot. In Victorian England, it was decided to publish only a few copies due to the fear the book would cause controversy in such an ultra-conservative society. The public at large did not enjoy the *Kama Sutra* until the '60s, eighty years later.

Below we will share the secrets of this classic Hindu text, but in an updated form which is designed to surprise your lover with exciting positions for oral sex.

The *Kama Sutra* gives a special place to kissing and licking particular areas of the body, an essential part of sexual play. The basic idea is to delay, for as long as possible, contact with the genitals and use foreplay to maximize excitation for the most intense orgasm possible. To do this, the lover must pay attention to other parts of the body such as the inner part of the thighs, the back of the knees, the breasts and nipples, the nape of the neck, ears, and abdomen, all of which prove to be highly eroto-genic areas.

To kiss and lick areas around the genitals, then suddenly move to other parts of the body, can serve as a very exciting strategy. It is also important to realize that each of these areas requires a different approach and, at times, the tongue's special attention. Since everyone reacts differently to stimulation, it's important to pay attention to the reactions of your partner—their movements and words which indicate, at any given moment, what they like or dislike.

The *Kama Sutra*, naturally, gives great importance to rub-bing and caresses. To rub your partner's skin or each other's genitals can be very pleasurable. Sometimes, just to notice the feel of your partner's erect nipples on your skin or, even better, to slide your own (covered with massage oil) over the pubic area of your partner is a sure-fire way to heat up the room. Pressure, also, is a very sensual tool. To press your bodies together, or press your partner against the wall with your hips joined can give rise to very erotic and satisfying sensations (especially in public places or situations where sex becomes something quickly furtive).

POSITIONS FOR CUNNILINGUS

Classic. This is when the man lies between the woman's legs, face down, or beside her, with his head level with her pelvis. In this position it is recommended that the woman have a pillow under her butt. This will make stimulating her clitoris easier and he can also avoid cramping his neck. This is the most comfortable position for cunnilingus and, to make it a bit more kinky, she can rest her head on a large pillow so she can "contemplate" the progress of her lover. To enjoy it better, she should keep her legs somewhat close, rather than fully open. This way, she'll be able to have more control over any movements of her pelvic muscles.

The key to any position of oral sex is comfort, especially when it comes to cunnilingus. Oral stimulation, for her, takes some time, and that's why it's important for both to adopt a relaxed posture which permits maximum freedom of movement. Some women will squeeze their legs together when they reach the critical point of excitation. If, in this moment, the man puts too much pressure on her, he can stifle and interrupt her climax. To avoid this, she should keep her knees bent and he should put his arms under the arch formed by her legs.

Another variation of this position is when the man lies on his back with the woman sitting on top of him, her knees on the sides of his shoulders, so that her genitals are right up against his face. This helps the man to get at her clitoris, as well as masturbate or stimulate her vulva with his fingers.

Standing. Subdue your guy; there is nothing more exciting to a couple. Undress, stand in front of him with your back against the wall, and make him kneel before you. Move your genitals close to his face, open your legs, and grab him (gently) by the hair and have him sink his mouth into you. If you have not tied his hands (an attractive alternative), you can have him massage your butt and the inner part of your thighs. Or, you can have him stimulate your clitoris with his fingers as his tongue works feverishly below, up and down, and make sure he changes the rhythm to your liking. In this position *you* have all the power and *he* must obey you!

SITTING...

- **On his face, facing him.** This position is a treat for both partners. On one hand, he is comfortably on his back with his mouth up and passive to you. On the other, you can control everything: speed, rhythm, and depth of stimulation. Sitting on him with your knees astride his shoulders, he can easily reach your "G" spot with his fingers, while you move at your own rhythm. He can also help by holding your waist to support your movements.

Your lover can also squeeze your butt or moisten his fingers with saliva and massage your nipples. The sight of your genital region in this position will be an added treat to your guy. This is possibly the most favorite position for men. Even so, it can be a bit tiring for the girl since she is taking all the initiative. For this approach, it is best for her to sit close to the headrest and use it to support her movements.

- **On his face, facing away from him.** This position allows him easy access to your clitoris and anus. The man can reach your butt cheeks and massage them, as well as stimulate your anus with his fingers.

- **On the edge of the bed.** In this position she sits on the edge of the bed with one leg bent while she offers her genitals to her lover. He is positioned on his knees in front of her.

Doggie-style. In this posture she has her forearms and knees on the bed and lifts her pelvis, offering her rump to her lover. He gets on his knees, behind her, and is able to stimulate her clitoris and anus at will.

This position gives the man total freedom of movement; he can stimulate this zone with his tongue, kiss her rump, massage her vulva. . . while she moves rhythmically in search of the best angle for pleasure. Doggy-style can be a bit tiring for the man, since he must maintain a bent-over posture for some while. To avoid cramps, he can lie down, from time to time, with his mouth up and continue stimulating her with his back supported by the mattress.

Legs on his shoulders. In this position, the woman lies on her back with her legs open and puts them over the man's shoulders, with her heels on his back. This provides very direct contact and allows the man to grab his partner's butt and push whenever he wants.

There are many variations of this basic position, but all have the man placed between her legs. And as with all instances when the man is between the woman's legs, he is able to provide great stimulation to the clitoris, or vagina, or the "G" spot with his fingers.

Remind your man at all times that your clitoris is very sensitive to direct stimulation and that he should go slowly, first caressing the hood which encircles it, kissing the inside of its folds, and always watching your reactions. If it is stimulated with too much pressure this can irritate or over-stimulate it, causing tension in the pelvic musculature and overloading the nerve endings, without giving any pleasure. And so it's important to pay close attention to the movements, utterances, or instructions of our partner so that we become aware of what gives her the most pleasure.

Thoroughly. She lies back with her legs open and lets her shoulders rest against his knees (she is facing him, sitting on his lap). The man places his hands under her rump and lifts her gently, drawing her crotch to his mouth.

This way he can deeply stimulate her clitoris, as well as her anus and perineum. She can drape her legs over her partner's shoulders and, inclined slightly forward, control the rhythm and depth of his cunnilingus.

All for me. This posture is one of the most exciting for a woman, in that she has total control over the movements and pressure and the man is totally at her command.

Here the woman sets herself upright on her knees on the mattress, legs apart. Her lover lies on his back with his mouth just underneath her vulva. This way, she can use a support (for example, the headrest of the bed) and control the movements of her pelvis so she gets maximum excitement. The man can grasp her waist and help her with the motion.

In this configuration, he can begin caressing the inner part of her thighs, and later continue by stimulating the perineum and anus, avoiding her vulva for the moment. This massage can be done with fingers, lips, or tip of the tongue. There is no need to hurry. He can use his hot breath all over her nether parts to make her melt.

This position is ideal for stimulating the anal sphincter and giving her a "black kiss" (more details later). With a finger in his lover's anus, the man can begin gently licking his partner's crotch and slowly approach the big lips of her vulva. He then opens his mouth and deeply kisses her Mount of Venus, with his tongue making its way to her clitoris.

In a chair. The truly exciting thing about oral sex is that you can practice it anywhere and make it as kinky as you want. Here is a way to enjoy it in the office, at home, on a solitary park bench, or in a hammock on the beach at dusk. With infinite possibilities, it is just a question of using a bit of imagination.

The woman should sit on the edge of a chair, easy chair, or hammock, etc., with legs open, offering herself to her lover. He should be on his knees between her legs and have one of her legs over his shoulder. This way, he has much deeper access with his mouth. He also has an exciting view of his partner's genitals and his hands are completely free to place them wherever he pleases.

Seated this way, he can start licking, kissing, and nibbling the inner part of her thighs. As he gets closer to her vulva, she will feel the heat of his approaching breath. He can also masturbate himself in this position with one of his free hands, further turning up the heat. Finally, the man brings his lips to her vulva and begins to kiss her voluptuously, brushing her clitoris, vibrating his tongue inside her, licking around her inner and outer lips. She can take her lover's head and move it to apply more pressure or change the rhythm, bringing more excitement as she reaches climax.

Legs up. In this position, the woman lies back on the mattress and holds her thighs, drawing her legs to her chest and offering her lover her entire genital area. He lies, face down, and sinks his mouth into her sex. His hands are free and he can grab her butt cheeks, rub her from top to bottom, and explore every nook and cranny of her body. This is also an ideal position to stimulate her anus and perineum.

She can grab her lover's head, stroke his hair, and draw him to her sexual part, as well as determine what pressure or rhythm excites her the most.

ADVICE FOR GUYS

The majority of men enjoy fellatio best of all. As soon as their lover brings her lips close to their genitals, they melt with pleasure. But when it comes time to return the favor, they often bail out.

Here are some tips for your guy to help him become a master of cunnilingus. Let him study these at length, so he can pay you back!

- **The majority of women** like stimulation of their clitoris to begin slowly and gently, progressing gradually and adding pressure bit by bit.
- **All movements** should always be done carefully but firmly.
- **Stroke delicately** from top to bottom when caressing the big and little lips of the vulva. Some women are mesmerized by rapidly moving the tongue over the vagina and then to the clitoris.
- **Give her a little massage** with licks or sucking; make sure to use different strokes. This will prevent the experience from becoming too monotonous.
- **Play,** using your nose, mouth, and chin so that you give her some variety.
- **Keep your beard** well shaved. Beard stubble irritates the vagina and is quite unpleasant.
- **Give her gentle, tender kisses** on her pubic hair until you arrive at her vagina's inner parts.
- **Nibble** her vaginal lips with great care.

- **With your tongue** in her vagina, use your fingers and introduce them, one by one, into the opening, penetrating gently and using a pulsing motion once inside. Remember to caress her breasts, too!
- **Breathe through your nose** carefully while inside her vagina as you massage its lips with your tongue.
- **When a woman has an orgasm,** her clitoris becomes a lot more sensitive, so don't go back on it immediately for oral sex, since this might hurt her.
- **Important Information.** Extreme sensitivity of the clitoris is a tip-off that orgasm has occurred. If you think it's a false alarm, however, touch her clitoris and watch her reaction. If she remains still, like nothing happened, you can be sure she hasn't climaxed yet.

The most important thing is to be sympathetic, affectionate, and sensitive. Cater to your lady's preferences; discover what turns her on.

THE 8 TECHNIQUES OF CUNNILINGUS, ACCORDING TO VATSYAYANA*

- **"ADHARA-SPHURITAM" (THE QUIVERING KISS).** With the tips of your fingers, gently pinch together the arched lips of her "house of love" very slowly, and kiss them as if you were kissing her lower lip.
- **"JIHVA-BHRAMANAKA" (THE CIRCLING TONGUE).** Spread apart the "vault" of her love nest with your nose. Let your tongue gently probe her yoni. Move your nose, lips, and chin, in circles.
- **"JIHVA-MARDITA" (THE TONGUE MASSAGE).** Let your tongue rest for a moment in the archway to the flower-adorned

"Lord's temple" before entering to worship vigorously, causing her juices to flow.

- **"CHUSHITA" (SUCKED).** Press your lips firmly on her vulva and suck hard on her clitoris.
- **"UCHCHUSHITA" (SUCKED UP).** Cup and lift up her buttocks. Let your tongue-tip probe her navel. Slither down to enter the archway of the love-god's dwelling and lap up her love-water.
- **"KSHOBAKA" (STIRRING).** Stirring the root of her thighs, which she keeps widely separated, your tongue drinks at her sacred spring.
- **"BAHUCHUSHITA" (SUCKED HARD).** With her feet on your shoulders, clasp her waist, suck hard, and let your tongue stir her overflowing love-temple.
- **"KAKILA" (THE CROW).** With both of you lying on your side, facing opposite ways, kiss each other's secret parts.

*Wise man and Hindu philosopher, author of the *Kama Sutra*

WHAT TYPE OF WOMAN ARE YOU?

Based on the depth of your yoni (vagina), the *Kama Sutra* tells us there are three types of women:

- **DEER WOMAN.** This type of woman has a yoni six fingers deep. Her body is delicate, almost infantile in appearance, smooth and tender. Her head is small and well-formed, her bust is erect, her belly is slender, and her thighs are fleshy. Her arms are long and rounded. She has thick, curly hair, black eyes, large cheeks, and big ears. She has an affectionate temperament with a quick mind, though, on occasion, she can be jealous.
- **MARE WOMAN.** This woman has a yoni nine fingers deep. Her body is delicate, but with sturdy arms. Her breasts are

large and her hips are wide. Her gait is graceful. She loves to sleep, and keeps her house neat. She is very affectionate with her partner.

- **ELEPHANT WOMAN.** The yoni of this type is twelve fingers deep. She has very big breasts. Her nose and ears are large and thick. She has very fleshy cheeks and lips. She has vigorous, black hair. Her feet, hands, and arms are short and rounded. It is more difficult to bring this woman to orgasm and one must make sure that coitus with her is long and slow.

POSITIONS FOR FELLATIO

Classic. This is the most comfortable and passive position for him. The man lies on his back with his legs open and knees slightly bent. The woman either reclines or kneels before him where she can have total control of the situation. She can kiss him over all his body, caress him, or masturbate him, going down seductively towards his genitals and "torturing" him, all the while delaying contact of her lips on them. If the man lies with pillows under his head, he will have an exciting "field of vision" for observing her.

Another variation of classic fellatio consists of tying (gently, with a handkerchief) the man's hands to the headrest of the bed and completely blindfolding him. In this submissive posture, she has complete control, with the man totally defenseless and at the mercy of every whim and desire of his partner. This is a very exciting situation for both partners who, later on, can exchange roles.

To obtain full erection, sucking and stimulation by the tongue must be continual. To bring him to orgasm, it is important to pace your rhythm with your partner's breathing, utterances, and involuntary movements. You can take his ejaculation in your mouth or anywhere else you desire. This always depends on the situation and desires of both partners.

Be aware that every man is different and responds in his own way to stimulation of his penis: to stroking, to pressure and to rhythm. You must pay attention to his face and other responses; you can also discuss it with him either before or afterwards. Ask him what he likes and how to give him the most stimulation.

You needn't follow everything you read in this book too literally. Let your imagination go and be spontaneous. Remember that your mental attitude is the most important factor when it comes to pleasure and mutual excitement.

Submissive lover. This is the favorite of most men since it allows them freedom of movement and an incomparable point of view with their lover at their feet. The man sits up with his legs apart and arms open to receive his lover. She begins to massage, to kiss, to lick his neck, chest, nipples. . . working her way down to his abdomen and navel. Her hands caress his thighs, his rump, etc. The man then gets on his feet, waiting for his lover to bring her hot lips to him and give him mind-altering fellatio.

After these preliminaries, she gets on her knees with her face level with his pubis. She then breathes on him seductively and plays with his testicles, not ceasing to stroke her guy's butt and thighs. This is when she takes the shaft of his penis and introduces it gently into her mouth. She begins to move, imitating coitus with her mouth, while her tongue stimulates his glans. She forms an "O" with her lips and circles the crown of his glans and the frenum, making circular movements.

She keeps his penis well-moistened with her saliva and makes sure he is constantly aware of her hot breath. Not forgetting the other senses, she looks up at him with eyes full of desire and gives seductive moans of pleasure.

This is a very active position for both partners. He can grab his lover's head and guide it to make her movements more pleasurable. Just be careful with this. Men get really excited in this position and are liable, when standing, to move as if they were having full-on coitus with their partner's mouth. Not being able to control the depth of his penetration, the man can easily gag his lover.

Another variety of this position is with the man standing as well, but supporting his butt on the edge of a table, bed, or easy-chair, while she sits on the floor (or better yet, on a pillow or cushion), half tilted, resting on one of her butt cheeks, with her knees bent. In this position she can begin to play with her lover's testicles while she firmly grasps the shaft of his penis. She runs her lips and tongue torridly over the surface of his foreskin and glans. Once it is well lubricated, she introduces it into her mouth and starts moving like it's coitus, but gently, slowly, gradually increasing the rhythm until he comes undone in ecstasy.

Remember, if your lover senses you are enjoying giving him fellatio, you are halfway to climaxing him. For that reason, you should add a little "juice" and not skimp on moans, little grunts, soft words. . . which set your boy's desire on fire. If he sees you turned on, that will turn *him* on even more!

On top of her. In this position she lies on her back with him straddling her with his knees on both sides of his lover's head.

This way, his penis is virtually on top of her lips and all she has to do is open her mouth to receive her lover's hot "gift."

For her, this is basically a passive position. But having her hands free, she can grab her lover's butt and pull him closer to her, simultaneously stimulating and massaging his thighs and even his anus.

This position allows deep penetration of the penis into her mouth, as well as one of the favorite fantasies of most men (and many women, too): ejaculating on her breasts or face.

On the knees. Both partners are on their knees on the bed and begin to stimulate each other. They give kisses, strokes, and nibbles to each other while each masturbates in front of the other. As this happens, she arches her back and approaches her lover's penis with her lips while continuing to stimulate her clitoris with the other hand.

This posture provides very deep oral stimulation. Meanwhile, he can stroke her hair, her face, her back, and even her breasts. Orgasm is sure to follow!

She's seated. This deals with a very seductive position and, above all, one that is very comfortable for her. The woman sits on the edge of the bed with open legs. He stands on the mattress and moves his penis towards his lover's mouth. While she is masturbating, he puts his penis into her hot mouth. With her other hand she can stimulate her partner's perineum and anus, or play with his testicles. She runs her mouth over his penis from top to bottom while he draws her mouth to him until he reaches climax.

The sexiest number. As the form of the numeral graphically illustrates, "69" allows each lover to stimulate the other's genitals in comfort and, best of all, simultaneously.

This position is so versatile that it is used not only for simultaneous oral sex, fellatio, and cunnilingus, but also can be alternated with techniques of genital masturbation or anal play. Often it is used as foreplay prior to penetration, but if the partners use appropriate stimulation it can also become a very pleasant way of reaching orgasm and ejaculation by itself.

In general, the woman lies on top of the man with her genitals in his face and her mouth on his penis (with the man on top it is somewhat more complicated for the woman to stimulate his erect penis).

There is, however, a position much more comfortable and relaxing for the two of them. It consists of both lying on their side, parallel to each other, genitals at the face of the other.

There are, in addition to 69, other numerals to consider such as 696, when we're talking about a threesome, or 6969, when talking about an orgy! Another exciting variation is 70 (69+1). In this case, the "+1" refers to the finger of one of the lovers introduced into the anus of the other.

Though 69 is a very exciting position, there are certain inconvenient aspects to it that you should keep in mind. For one thing, while each lover is being orally stimulated, it often occurs that one of them gets sidetracked because of the pleasure they are receiving. This can result in forgetting to pleasure the other sufficiently. One way to avoid this "lapse" is to keep the inverted position, and while one of them orally stimulates their partner, the other masturbates the first, later exchanging roles. This way it is much easier for both to reach orgasm together.

In this position, maneuvering of hands is substantially reduced and using the tongue to reach the clitoris is also more complicated.

EVEN IN THE CAR...

We've already noted that you can have oral sex anytime, anywhere. The automobile is a classic place for oral sex, and here we offer the most exciting positions for doing it "on the fly."

- **FROM LEFT TO RIGHT.** He sits in the driver's seat and she leans towards him from the passenger side.
- **FROM BEHIND.** He kneels between the two front seats, facing towards the rear, and puts his penis in the space between them. She engages in oral sex from the back seat.
- **69.** Both lovers are in the rear seat. She is on the bottom with her legs open, and he is on all fours on top of her, in the opposite orientation.
- **WITH THE DOOR OPEN.** With the door open, either one sits in whatever seat they like, with the other partner outside on their knees, giving the "inside" partner oral sex.

WHAT TYPE OF MAN ARE YOU?

According to the *Kama Sutra*, a man may be classified according to the size of his lingam (penis):

- **THE RABBIT.** He has a lingam which does not exceed six fingers in length when erect. It is said he is a short man, but with a well-formed body. His hands, knees, feet, and thighs are small. He has a round face, small, fine teeth, silky hair and big, open eyes. He has a calm temperament; he desires fame, though he is humble. He is abstemious in eating and moderate in all his carnal desires.
- **THE BULL.** When erect, his penis measures nine fingers in length. His body is robust and solid, broad-chested, rock-bellied. His forehead is wide and his eyes are large. He has a restless, irascible temperament.

- **THE HORSE.** This one comes with a twelve-finger erection. He is tall, but not heavy. He prefers big, robust women. He has a hard body with a wide, muscular chest. His teeth, neck, and ears are big, as are his hands and fingers. His hair is thick, his look is determined and hard, and his voice is deep. His is daring, passionate, and ambitious of spirit.

Red Hot!

You should be clear about one thing: sex is all in the mind. If you are imaginative, fun, curious, and daring, your lover is in luck. The secret is to free yourself and dare to try new things without fear or repression. Let your erotic imagination go; dive into sexual fantasy and fire up your sexual energy and power of seduction. Leave all limits behind and let exciting ideas and dreams inspire how you make love with your partner. Remember that guilt makes for poor sex. Everything you do in sex is OK, as long as it is done with a free spirit, treasuring every moment.

Make sure you put your fantasies into play. Throw out shame, false modesty, and taboos. Sex is one of the most liberating and pleasing activities a human being can enjoy. Don't put limits on your sexuality; let yourself go in total confidence and all naturalness.

To this end it is important to share with your partner. Tell him or her your sexual fantasies without leaving out any of the details and let them know that you want to share them with him or her. Get your lover to tell you their fantasies too; it is likely you have more than a few in common. This sharing is the main ingredient for a healthy, sincere, and frank relationship, and the ideal recipe for turning up the heat on your mutual desire.

INDECENT PROPOSALS

There are many ways you can share your "perversions" with your lover, the ones which fire up your desire. In previous chapters we have talked about foreplay. There is no reason you have to wait until you are in bed to start foreplay; you can begin to "warm up the engine" even at the office. Send your partner some sexy text messages, something risqué in tone that will get them going the rest of the day, fantasizing about what you're going to do when you get them alone. You can be sure this seductive, unexpected little incitement will pique their desire. And if you want to use a more direct approach, you can always call them on the telephone. Fill your partner's head with exciting images, whisper dirty little nothings, and promise them you're serious about sharing those fantasies that really get them going.

BREAKFAST IN BED

We are not talking about your typical buttered toast and orange juice. Wake a bit earlier than usual and slip your hands under the sheets. Slowly, sweetly, start to caress her "little treasure" with moistened fingertips. The idea is to make her come without waking her up. Well, almost. (By the way, this practice is known as somnophilia.) Don't open the window, turn on the lights, or make any sudden movements. She has to feel like she is having an erotic dream. Go down on her and give her a gentle morning session of oral sex. If it's the weekend, you can go on to coitus, but if she's got to go to work, stop before that; remind her she owes you and you want it back later, with interest. You will see how your lover remembers every detail of her kinky reveille all through the day and how she won't be able to wait till nighttime to settle the account with you!

THE "BLACK KISS"

The anus is a very erotic zone, but many couples have reservations about including it in a session of oral sex. Know that as far as men are concerned, the proximity of the prostate to the anus makes it an extremely pleasurable area, if it is stimulated properly. Just remember, this can be a touchy subject and many men feel their masculinity is threatened when this "off-limits" zone is handled.

For starters, you can give him a gentle massage around his anus with moistened fingers. Spend some time doing this as you fondle his testicles with your other hand. Use a gentle touch, natural, without forcing it. Ask him, from time to time, if he likes it and if what you're doing excites him. His groans, his facial expression, and his words will tell you if you should keep on going or stop and go to another area. If your guy is up to it, continue by putting your finger in a bit deeper and move it in a circular movement, carefully. Obviously, anal sex requires some basic hygiene for hands and rear-end.

If you want, you can make your way between his butt cheeks with your hot tongue while you stimulate his penis with your hand.

The "black kiss" or anallingus (oral stimulation of the anus) is an exciting complement to fellatio and cunnilingus. The ideal position for success is to get down on all fours and let your lover place him-/herself behind you with their head below the arch formed by your legs. That way, they can stimulate and lick the entire anal and genital area, as well as play with your rump and the inner part of your thighs.

At first, the rectal area responds to stimulation by contracting. For this reason it's important your partner relaxes and feels comfortable with your explorations of their rear before you put your tongue there. Massage their back and butt; kiss and rub the front of their thighs. Carefully lick, suck, and nibble their rump, perineum, and the skin around their anus. Warm up and moisten the area with your mouth.

The rectum contracts when first stimulated, and then it expands. Lick it or touch it with the tip of your tongue, and watch its response. The muscles of the sphincter will begin to relax, allowing you to explore it deeper.

Using fingers is a very exciting way to stimulate the anal zone. The vagina shares a wall with the rectum and a series of erogenous zones as well, along with many nerve endings. You can alternate manual stimulation with licks and kisses (watch out: use great caution and do this only when the area is sufficiently excited and dilated). Moisten or lubricate a finger and start by stroking the anal opening. Carefully, gradually, introduce the finger until it touches the "G" spot (refer to the chapter on orgasm). Stimulate it with little circles and by moving the finger up and down.

A final piece of advice: oral stimulation of the anus requires certain precautions. Keep in mind the presence of certain bacteria that live in the large intestine and colon which can cause infection. So if you want to do the "black kiss," practice extremely good hygiene and be sure you know the person with whom you're doing it.

For his pleasure. Have him get down on all fours and lie on your back with your head beneath his legs. Start sucking his penis while you moisten your fingers in your vagina or with saliva. Play with his ass cheeks and don't stop licking him as you begin to stimulate his perinuem (the area between the base of his testicles and anus) with light and gentle pressure.

Now, get on your knees, behind your lover, and begin by dragging your tongue along the crack of his butt. Let your hot breath stimulate the whole area as you continue to masturbate his penis with your other hand. Moisten one of your fingers with saliva and massage the outer ring of his anus. The idea is, bit by bit, for him to get used to your stimulation. As his excitement increases, open his ass cheeks and kiss between them, lick his anus, and push it with the tip of your tongue. Stimulate his perineum with one hand as you continue to masturbate him with the other, until he comes.

Don't forget about his testicles, how sensitive and capable they are of reacting to the slightest touch. The skin of the scrotum is delicate and when stroked produces very pleasant sensations. Just holding the testicles makes for something very pleasant. Support them gently, but firmly, in your hand. This always gives rise to a delicious effect, which spreads to the entire genital area. Stimulating the scrotum also arouses the surrounding area.

Another pleasant way to stimulate the testicles is to slide your fingertips over the scrotum and give them a gentle massage. A firm massage with the tip of your tongue at the base of his penis also produces intense, but pleasing sensations.

During fellatio, it is exciting to forget the penis for a while and give his testicles their due. You can kiss, lick—making small circles with the tongue-tip—or nibble (careful: just the skin which surrounds them).

And remember that most-erogenous zone that lies behind the testicles: the perineum. Stimulate it with your fingertips, run your tongue over it, press it gently.

For her pleasure. Same position, but it is now she who is on all fours and he who lies under her legs. Enjoy yourself as you lick her vulva and clitoris with your hot tongue. Massage her butt cheeks and put your fingers in the crease between them. Keep licking her perineum and gently rub the outside of her anus to make her rectal area relax.

Kiss her ass cheeks, making concentric spirals from outside to inside. Stretch your tongue and move it close to the outer part of her anus. Press with the tip and move gently towards the inner part. Stimulate her clitoris until she reaches climax.

CHANGE OF SCENERY

We've already commented how monotony and lack of imagination are the worst enemies of sex. As exciting as your sexual escapades may be, you can always top them with a little something extra, perhaps a "kinky" touch that fires up the passion of the moment. One of the great advantages, and pleasures, of oral sex is that you can do it virtually anywhere and in any situation. So don't limit yourself at home by just doing it in the comfort of your bed. Try out the bathroom, the kitchen, the living room sofa, or the deckchair on the terrace.

If you have a stairway, why not give it a try? Steps are ideal for oral sex due to their difference in level. Just sit on the stairs (you'll be more comfortable if you use cushions), with your partner's head between your legs and their knees on a lower step. This will allow better mobility of their head.

Every place has its "kinky" aspect, if we only let our imagination soar. There are endless possibilities for greater excitement. You can do it outdoors. The element of risk involved in doing it in public, where someone might surprise you, adds an exciting twist for many couples. It is the celebrated "quickie" hookup, which can be enjoyed as an incredible session of oral sex in the office, in your car, on a deserted beach, the fitting room in a clothing store, or the public restroom of a restaurant.

HOW TASTY!

Oral sex is a practice that gives rise to a lot of prejudgments and inhibitions. One of the most common concerns revolves around the color and taste of the genitals, as well as their secretions. There is nothing better to chase away those "phantoms" than to propose a romantic and exciting shared bath. You can add to the level of seduction of your bath by incorporating rose petals, scented candles, essential oils, and bathing salts.

If the taste of oral sex continues to be a problem, you can buy any number of sexual lubricants specially designed for this pleasure. They are completely edible and are available in luscious flavors such as strawberry, lemon, mint, chocolate, etc. You can also use extra-strong mint candy while you suck on his penis (he will enjoy this too) or put a capsule of edible sexual lubricant in your mouth and crack it open with your teeth. Another option is to use toothpaste (this gives a sensation of freshness) or even a shot of cognac (sensation of heat).

There's an injunction: "Don't play with your food." This time, however, we will leave this wise counsel and use food as an ideal condiment to spice up our session of oral sex. Ingredients such as whipped cream, marmalade, champagne, honey, yogurt, chocolate, or wine allow us to further "savor" our lover's body.

Here are some tasty recipes:

- Slowly pour a trickle of sparkling rose wine on your lover's Mount of Venus. Let the little stream of bubbly descend to her vagina and meet it there with your tongue. Lick the lips, the clitoris… drink the refreshing vintage from the most sensuous cup imaginable.

- Prepare thick hot chocolate and let it cool down a while in a bowl. Add a few tablespoons of whipped cream. With a brush, spread this delicacy on the navel and genitals of your lover. Let your greedy tongue enjoy the sweet banquet: sip it, lick it, suck it, devour it totally, with pleasure…

- Mix strawberry yogurt with a bit of honey. Let it chill in the refrigerator, and use it to garnish her clitoris. Spread it smoothly in small amounts so that it slides over the hood of her clitoris and little lips of her vulva. Do this very slowly so that the chill stimulates the area and later you can lick her, greedily!

• Freshen up his penis with some mint. Rinse your mouth with the strongest mouthwash you can find, or take a super-strong mint candy and give him refreshing fellatio. Your mentholated tongue will give him new, fresh experiences due to its properties as a vasoconstrictor.

• Don't forget to have a box of scented wipes available so you can clean up (both of you) after the banquet!

GOOD VIBRATIONS

Surely you must have heard about the ring vibrator used to stimulate the clitoris during penetration. These are placed at the end of the shaft of the penis and small batteries make it vibrate during coitus.

The sex toy industry now offers a novelty, which provides exciting and pleasurable sessions of oral sex. The device in question is a ring vibrator, which is put on the tongue (available in several sizes and colors) and gives much more intense oral stimulation for both the man and the woman.

DOUBLE YOUR PLEASURE

If you have an open-minded and free relationship with your partner, you can always go one step beyond in your sexual encounters. We're talking about including a third person in your oral sex play. This is the star-attraction fantasy of every man: to have sex with two women at the same time. For women, this fantasy is usually to have sex with two men, but there are those who prefer that one of the two partners be another woman.

If you are able to overcome bashfulness or cultural inhibitions, this "round robin" of pleasure can turn into something very exciting.

For example, in multiple oral sex, one of the women can give the other woman cunnilingus, while the second licks the man's penis. They can take turns, or else give the man fellatio together while they swap off masturbating him. One can suck on his glans, while the other strokes the root of his penis from top to bottom. Then one of them can lick his scrotum, while the other takes his penis in her mouth and sucks him for all it's worth. On this point in common, which is the man's penis, they might end up kissing each other or having their tongues entwined—a lesbian-conjuring image which greatly excites men.

In the case of two men and one woman, she has two penises to play with, and even better, two tongues which can give her an unforgettable session of cunnilingus. She can give fellatio to one while she masturbates the other.

She can play with both penises on her lips and even lick them together at the same time, glans against glans. When it is her time to receive, she can get down on all fours and let them stimulate her vagina, her perineum, her anus… in an irresistible clash of tongues and hot breath. Or, in this position, she can give one of them fellatio while the other gives her cunnilingus as he lies on his back between her legs.

THE MOST SENSUAL PIERCING

Piercing goes far beyond simple esthetics. Done on certain parts of the body, it can be the perfect way to increase sexual pleasure. It can aid stimulation of the genitals, above all the clitoris, if it is located there. Most women pierce either their *labia minora*, at the bottom of the vaginal opening, or the perineum. These piercings are very sensual, and to play with those in the nipples as well as the genitals can be very exciting.

Even so, one must take every precaution not to engage in positions that can result in injury, and, regarding hygiene, make sure to avoid infections.

Daring places to have piercings include: nipples, tongue (very exciting for giving your guy fellatio), or clitoris. A piercing in the navel is less "hardcore," but very erotic anyway.

If you get a piercing in your tongue, your lover will experience a windfall of pleasure when you give him oral sex. Since a piercing is metallic, it is an excellent conductor of heat and provides you with a tool you can use to intensify or vary the stimulation you give in oral sex. A good idea is drinking something hot or cold prior to putting your mouth on your partner's penis or vulva. The piercing will retain the temperature of the beverage, and this will be much more seductive and sensual for your lover.

Make sure to engage the services of a professional when you get pierced and that the level of hygiene is the same you would expect at a dentist's office. This is to avoid the risk of infection or other sickness such as hepatitis or AIDS.

Keep your "little jewels" clean at all times. Wash them in hot water and neutral soap after every sexual encounter. Avoid soaps that are too strong or overly perfumed.

DECORATE YOURSELF!

Forget about clothes for a second and surprise your partner with a new look in nudity: body painting! You can do it yourself at home or go to a professional who can trim you from top to bottom. The paints used for this have been adapted for use on the skin so as to avoid any allergic reactions or irritation. They come in different colors and tastes, which your partner can lick in suggestive and sensual ways.

HOW ABOUT A SHOWER?

If you enjoy trying out new spots with your partner, why not try oral sex in the shower? We've already talked about the necessity of good hygiene before oral sex. Here we are going to combine the two: personal hygiene and pleasure!

Before you start, why don't you spruce up the bathroom a bit? Usually somewhat cold and impersonal, you can give this space an erotic touch and make it more sensual with candles, incense, and sultry music. Be careful and make sure the wiring for the sound equipment is as far as possible from water so you don't get shocked.

The temperature of the space is also important. Take into account that you are naked and getting splashed with water, so make sure the bathroom is well heated.

Now that you've taken care of the setting, it's time for action. Both of you get in the shower and let the hot water run over your nude skin. For her, it is especially erotic to direct the stream of water directly on the vagina. This is very sensual and exciting. In the meantime, your partner can soap your back and run his slippery hands over your butt, your breasts, your abdomen, etc. He can start to explore your more intimate areas with his moistened fingers and slowly, but surely, heat up the shower even more.

The essential thing is to let go, to enjoy yourselves, to experience the hot water and foam, and, above all, to talk to each other. Tell him what you like and what you don't like so you can make it the best experience possible.

Each can also pleasure him- or herself, alone. It is extremely hot to watch your partner masturbating.

Turn off the water and push your guy's head down. Have him get down on his knees and have him "drink" your soaking genitals. Be careful not to slip. If the shower is not big enough you might have to hold on to one of the fixtures to steady yourself. Let him sink his face between your legs. To provide for deeper stimulation of his tongue, drape one of your legs over his shoulder.

Oral sex in the shower can sometimes be a little uncomfortable. Change positions to avoid any tiring, and little by little both can reach a nice, "soft-boiled" orgasm!

NAUGHTY PHONE SEX

In general, ladies love to spend time glued to the phone. Take advantage of this with your partner and give her a session of "opportunistic" phone sex. While she's chatting away, kneel in front of her, remove her shoes, and start kissing her feet, sensually. Don't tickle her or your presence will be tipped off to the other person on the line. Go up her legs with your kisses, making sure to rub against her skin. If she is wearing a skirt it will be easier for you to reach your "objective." If she happens to be wearing pants, unzip them quickly and surely.

Don't take no for an answer. If you manage to remove her clothes waist down, without any opposition, gently slide your fingertips over her nude skin. Start kissing the inside of her thighs and slowly approach her sexual part with your hot breath. Don't hurry. If you are too rough, you might cause her to interrupt her conversation with little moans or a change of voice which can betray your activity to her interlocutor. Once she's finished with the phone conversation you needn't get up; just finish what you started.

You also can use the telephone for the following game. Call a phone sex number (they're listed in the newspaper or Internet). If you have a speaker phone, use it; that will allow your free hands more exciting options and both of you will be able to share the sensual moment.

Have your guy do the talking and let him get excited from the fantasies the phone sex operator gives him. As things start heating up, unzip his pants and start to kiss, suck, and lick his penis. The greatest excitement will be generated if you are able to synchronize what you are doing to him with what is going on with the phone sex. And don't worry about the phone bill. Normally, phone sex fantasies get them going really quick and before you know it, he'll already have shot his dice!

DEEP THROAT

It was 1972 when Linda Lovelace became the sex icon of the day. Directed by Gerard Damiano (owner of a beauty parlor before he got into movie-making), *Deep Throat* told the story of a woman who couldn't reach orgasm during coitus because her clitoris, due to an unusual birth defect, was located in her throat! The film caused considerable uproar, both social and political. The Nixon administration launched an aggressive campaign to prevent distribution of the film, which unleashed a firestorm of controversy. The movie was banned in twenty-three states, and its protagonists were charged with "conspiracy to transport obscene materials across state lines."

Today, fortunately, times have changed and no one, or almost no one, is scandalized by these things. And so this legendary flick has inspired us to show you how to enjoy one of the most surprising and pleasing techniques of fellatio you can give to your lover.

It is not the easiest of positions to pull off. The secret lies in being able to breathe through your nose. You have to practice until you are able to completely control each part of its execution. If you are patient, you will see it was more than worth it once you see your guy's face after you have given him the best orgasm of his life!

As we've already said, to begin to train for this you must learn to breathe through your nose. Practice a while until you feel completely comfortable doing it. Now comes the hard part. You must be able to control the natural "gagging" reflex. You can start by introducing two or three fingers into your throat. Start off shallow, then go deeper gradually as you learn to better control the reflex. Try to keep your fingers in the back of your throat for four to five seconds. Meanwhile, keep breathing through the nose and RELAX. Remove your fingers, rest a moment, and then try again. You'll see, after a few days, with the help of nasal breathing the gagging reflex will start to disappear. Remember, this technique requires a lot of practice and mental focus.

The best "deep throat" position is to be on your knees with your shoulders arched backwards. Separate your knees, but keep your ankles together and hold them with your hands. Let your head roll back; this way your mouth and throat will be perfectly aligned and this will facilitate deep penetration of his penis.

Another position for deep throat is to lie down with your shoulders flat on the bed and let your head hang over the edge. This way you can make your neck and mouth align and allow superb oral penetration.

In both positions, he will have to place himself in front of your face. Have him hold you at the nape of your neck, so he can support your head and keep your mouth and throat in a straight line. You'll probably feel, at least the first few times, that he is choking you with his penis. Just remember your breathing exercises and focus your mind on the orgasm he will have. Tell your lover not to make any rough movements and, above all, not to force penetration.

TWO FOR THE PRICE OF ONE

It will drive your lover wild if you give him both oral and penetrating sex together. He will go nuts when you massage his penis, passing it from your mouth to your vagina, and then back again to your mouth. You should adopt a comfortable position that allows you freedom of movement. Know that you're going to move a lot and it is best if he lies on the bed face up with you on top.

Begin by sinking your mouth between his legs. Lick his penis for a while, then sit on his face and let him play a bit with your "inner parts." Let him stay there a couple of minutes, then take away your face. Sit on his pelvis and have him penetrate you. Don't let him get too deep into you; let him experience your heat a bit and then go back to his face for more oral sex. This switching from top to bottom will make him mad with pleasure, and you'll be the one who decides how it ends up!

ORAL TANTRA

Oral Tantric sex is a slow, sensual practice that can last hours.

According to the ancient tradition of Tantra, there are two positions for oral sex:

- **The "Kakasana" Position.** In this position, the woman (Shakti) and the man (Shakta) lie parallel to each other on their right sides with faces opposite the other's genitals. Shakta (the man) slips his right hand under the woman's thighs and rests his head between them. Then he moistens his thumb and index finger of his right hand with saliva and seals her anus with the index finger while he puts his thumb in her yoni (vagina). Then he rests his mouth on her yoni and starts to activate her clitoris with his tongue.

For her part, the Shakti sucks his lingam with her mouth, sealing off its opening with her tongue and pressing on his anus with the third finger of her right hand. She uses the rest of her fingers to massage his scrotum and perineum.

This position, called "Kakasana," brings about a gentle orgasm and allows the merging of the awareness of the "god" and "goddess" into a realm of transcendent peace.

- **Crow Position.** This is a complicated position, which requires great strength on the part of the man. The man stands while the woman wraps her legs around him, she being suspended in the air. He puts his mouth on her yoni and starts to activate her clitoris while she takes his penis in her mouth. This posture is used as a means to channel intense sexual energy.